Corneal Biomechanics and Refractive Surgery

Fabio A. Guarnieri

Editor

Corneal Biomechanics and Refractive Surgery

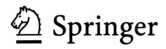 Springer

Editor
Fabio A. Guarnieri, PhD
Department of Bioengineering
Centro de Investigación de Métodos Computacionales (CIMEC)
Predio CONICET-Santa Fe, Colectora Ruta Nac 168, Km 472, Paraje El Pozo
3000 Santa Fe, Argentina

ISBN 978-1-4939-1766-2   ISBN 978-1-4939-1767-9 (eBook)
DOI 10.1007/978-1-4939-1767-9
Springer New York Heidelberg Dordrecht London

Library of Congress Control Number: 2014953899

Printed on acid-free paper

Springer is part of Springer Science+Business Media (www.springer.com)

Contents

Contributors

Paulo Ferrara Paulo Ferrara Eye Clinic, Keratoconus Unit, AV Contorno, B. Serra, Belo Horizonte, MG, Brazil

Fabio A. Guarnieri Department of Bioengineering, Centro de Investigación de Métodos Computacionales (CIMEC), Santa Fe, Argentina

Andrés Guzmán Universidad del Norte, Barranquilla, Atlantico, Colombia

Leonardo Torquetti Center for Excellence in Ophthalmology, Anterior Segment, RUA Capitão Teixeira, B. Nossa Senhora das Graças, Pará de Minas, MG, Brazil

Chapter 1
Introduction: Corneal Biomechanics and Refractive Surgery

Fabio A. Guarnieri

1 Refractive Surgery

This book is related to corneal biomechanics but stresses its importance to Refractive Surgery, an outstanding procedure that changed the way ophthalmologists and patients see ophthalmology.

The Refractive Surgery (RS) is a technique used in ophthalmology which modifies the refractive state of the eye. Since the cornea is the main responsible for the refraction of the eye, because its refractive power is greater than 70 % of the eye, its refractive properties are used to change the optical system of the eye. The RS is used in the correction of refractive errors like myopia, astigmatism, and farsightedness. Among other procedures of RS include radial and astigmatic keratotomy, photorefractive keratectomy, and keratomileusis.

Photorefractive keratectomy performs a molding of the cornea with short-wavelength (e.g., excimer 193 nm) laser. In this case it is assumed that the intraocular pressure does not affect the structure due to the low thickness of cornea removed. Keratomileusis is a procedure created by Jose Barraquer (Santa Fe de Bogota, Colombia) where an autograft is done, before casting it. A microkeratome is used to cut a sheet of cornea and with the excimer laser being mold in situ (LASIK).

Incisional surgery was the first surgical procedure approved by the FDA (Food and Drug Administration, USA) and has been clinically validated for over 15 years. Radial keratotomy and astigmatic keratotomy (RK and AK) are based on relaxing cuts with scalpel of diamond on the cornea, with maximum depth, without reaching perforation. Refractive change is achieved when the intraocular pressure relaxed

F.A. Guarnieri, Ph.D. (✉)
Department of Bioengineering, Centro de Investigación de Métodos
Computacionales (CIMEC), Predio CONICET-Santa Fe, Colectora Ruta Nac 168,
Km 472, Paraje El Pozo, 3000 Santa Fe, Argentina
e-mail: aguarni@santafe-conicet.gov.ar

© Springer Science+Business Media New York 2015
F.A. Guarnieri (ed.), *Corneal Biomechanics and Refractive Surgery*,
DOI 10.1007/978-1-4939-1767-9_1

1

Fig. 1.1 A diagram of a
radial keratotomy with four
incisions and the effect of
the intraocular pressure.
The cornea bends in the
incised area and flattens in
the not-incised center

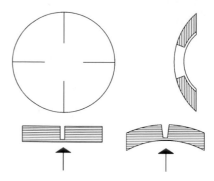

the corneal surface, increasing the curvature where the thickness is lower and
flattening the rest. In case of myopia and astigmatism it is intended that the central
or optics of the cornea to flatten. This is accomplished, for example, by making
radial cuts in the periphery of the optic zone, located inside a circle of diameter
approximately 3 mm (Fig. 1.1).

The history of the RK is outlined as follows:

- In the late nineteenth century, Snellen, Bates, and Lans made the first observations on the effect of RK.
- In 1930, Sato experimented in the laboratory and clinically with up to
  40 incisions.
- In 1970, Fyodorov and Durnev designed a multifactorial formula with an optical
  area greater than 3 mm in diameter.
- In 1978, Bores, Myers, and Cowden introduced the surgical technique in
  the USA.   ,
- In 1980, the NEI (National Eye Institute) of the USA conducted a prospective
  study in 9 clinical centers, yielding results in 1 and 3 years.

Since then several studies have been published based on different clinical nomograms (or diagrams of cuts), performed by several surgeons. Among them stand out
those from Ruiz et al. [1]. The aim, later, was to use a few and shorter incisions,
attempting to get minimally invasive procedures [2].

The calculation of the cuts in the RK and AK is mainly done by tables compiled
by surgeons depending on cases [3, 4]. Some techniques incorporate closed mathematical formulas based on simple models [3]. Both of them exhibit a lack of
prediction [4–6] because they do not consider the intrinsic behavior of the cornea
[7] or the biomechanics of the cornea. Table 1.1 shows the results of three studies of
RK, showing the percentage of eyes within the error of refraction [5].

The PERK study (Prospective Evaluation of Radial Keratotomy) [6] found that a
surgeon could only be secured with a 90 % certainty that the refraction of a patient
1 year after having surgery is within 1.75 D (diopters, refractive power) of the
predicted value. With regard to stability it was found that after a follow-up of
6 months to 4 years, the percentage of eyes with refractive change greater than

Table 1.1 RK clinical studies

	Estudio PERK (%)	Arrowsmith and Marks	Deitz and Sanders
±1.00 D	69	48 %	84 %
±1.50 D	86	–	94 %
±2.00 D	95	78 %	–

one diopter was 28 %. The study enhanced the importance of preoperative variables on the outcome of surgery. It found that the main factors are the diameter of central clear area, age of the patient, and the depth of the incision. According to this statistical study, patient gender, initial keratometric power, corneal thickness, corneal diameter, intraocular pressure, and ocular rigidity did not have great influence.

Binder et al. [8] demonstrated, through a study with electron microscopy and histochemistry, that the incision was healed completely only after 5 years of surgery. The excess time of scarring caused by steroids was attributed for the slow healing. The study described the changes in the scar in the incision, possible causes of fluctuating vision and progressive hyperopia.

These techniques can leave the patient with significant overcorrections or undercorrections. This lack of accuracy is due to calculation methods that do not include the complexity of the cornea. With the incorporation of digital videokeratoscopy [9], the corneal topography has been adequately represented, especially after a surgical procedure. Furthermore, other studies have been performed about corneal anisotropy [10] and viscoelasticity [11]. Other studies need to confirm the influence on the outcome of the RS because of the sclera, ocular muscles, optic nerve, and eyelid.

2   Biomedical Engineering

Biomedical Engineering is an interdisciplinary science between medicine and engineering. It was originally conceived for the development of medical equipment. However, in these days, it covers a wide range of activities, from the theoretical analysis of physiological processes to the practical design of unconventional therapies. In this line, computer models have been useful in understanding the mechanics of physiological processes. These models are used to simulate changes in these processes, for example, when they are affected by medical therapies.

Biomechanics is the study of the mechanics of biological systems [12]. In the human body, it helps to understand their normal function, to predict changes due to alteration, and to propose methods of artificial intervention. Its history is ancient. Aristotle, Leonardo Da Vinci, Newton, Descartes, and Helmholtz have made contributions to it. Problems such as the analysis of human movement for rehabilitation, sports, and surgery are of great interest in this area.

Computational Mechanics formulates methods and algorithms to investigate complex mechanical processes. They can undertake various analyses (structural, fluid dynamics, thermal, electromagnetic) based on the discretization of the continuum and can be applied different computational approaches such as finite element, finite volume, and boundary element methods, among others.

In last decades, medical researchers and engineers have begun to introduce predictive computational tools in medical practice. The aim is to use advanced simulation techniques, together with the powerful computational resources currently investigating the biomechanical behavior and ultimately improving and anticipating the results of medical procedures. Computational Biomechanics, branch of Biomechanics and Computational Mechanics, has become important in medical specialties such as orthopedics and cardiology. In orthopedics, it has improved hip [13], knee, and foot prostheses through the simulation. In cardiology there has been performed simulations of blood flow through valves [14], stenosis, arterial bifurcations [15], bypasses, etc. In ophthalmology, there have been some computational studies for research, especially in the RS, for the estimation of elastic parameters (see Chap. 2) and simulation of surgical procedures on the cornea (see Chaps. 3–5).

3   Biomechanical Models for Refractive Surgery

The procedures and principles of mechanical engineering, to achieve a mathematical model of the eye and the cornea, can provide help in studying the biomechanics of it and predict their behavior.

Early biomechanical studies on the cornea were oriented to its rheology (Chap. 2). Several mathematical models or theories have been proposed [3, 9, 16] using closed equations. Its reliability has been limited due to the aforementioned complexity of the cornea.

The cornea may be considered as a structure under pressure (atmospheric at the anterior surface, intraocular on the posterior surface), bounded to another structure having different characteristics such as the sclera. Obtaining the structural parameters of the material (Young's modulus, Poisson constant, relaxation times, etc.), the acting forces (intraocular pressure, effects of the eyelid, etc.), and geometry (thicknesses and topography), it is possible to perform a structural analysis using the finite element method.

The radial cuts of radial keratotomy can be simulated by modifying the geometry and by changing structural parameters like the healing material. The geometry obtained after the structural analysis is processed to monitor the optical effects and determine whether the surgical plan is correct.

To ensure that a corneal biomechanical model imitates the real behavior under the influence of the incisions (or under any other forces or geometric change, such as laser ablation or intrastromal implants) is necessary to determine their structural parameters. The bibliography is extensive in the description of the procedures and principles to determine the biomechanics of the cornea. Some authors consider that the cornea behaves as a linear elastic and isotropic material. Others go so far as to consider it as nonlinear, viscoelastic, and anisotropic (Chap. 2).

In order to build a complete biomechanical model, it is important to obtain the complete geometry of the cornea, both anterior and posterior curvature, and thicknesses, which vary from the optical center to the periphery. New technology exists for measuring such specific geometrical parameters: the digital videokeratoscope or corneal topographer, which determines the curvature of the anterior surface and the corneal pachymeter.

The benefits of applying computational methods in the RS, as well as other procedures, are immediate. The ophthalmologist (or bioengineer expert in ophthalmology) could perform countless iterations, under a wide range of circumstances, very quickly, with low investment of time and energy risk. It could perform a variety of operations on the computer to determine the parameters of surgery for each patient and achieve the desired refractive effect. In turn the patient with refractive problems would get higher reliability on these types of surgical procedures, preventing further surgeries or the use of low-grade glasses because of under- or overcorrections.

There is still a long way to this goal because it can only be estimated the constitutive parameters of the cornea and there is little information about the viscoelastic response and scar tissue from the cornea. Still, quantitative changes can be predicted with an accuracy comparable to that of standard calculation procedures and to investigate new nomograms and observe changes that would occur in a patient.

The development of computerized biomechanical models [thesis] saves time and resources, as the sacrifice of animals, allowing researching and implementing methods of diagnosis and correction of refractive eye diseases.

4   Chapter Organization

Chapter 2 presents a summary of the rheology and biomechanics of the corneal tissue and sclera. We present experimental work of various authors on obtaining mechanical parameters of the cornea such as scleral rigidity, elastic modulus, Poisson constant, anisotropy, viscoelasticity, tissue hydration, etc. It also described a summary of the mathematical models which simulate the refractive surgery and methods of data acquisition and processing.

In Chap. 3 the biomechanics of corneal tissue and a finite element model is applied to simulate incisional surgery like radial keratotomy (RK). An accurate geometric representation of the cornea is acquired with a digital videokeratoscope and an ultrasonic paquimeter. The simulation results are analyzed through a topographic map of the modified cornea. A parametric study and comparison with clinical results are discussed.

Chapter 4 describes investigation of the biomechanical response of the cornea to ALK, PRK, and LASIK using a computational modeling approach. The model provides data on the deformations of the stromal bed and may be used to predict the refractive outcome of surgery.

In Chap. 5 the biomechanical model is applied and modified to account the interaction of Ferrara ring segments in astigmatic and keratoconic eyes. It also described the biomechanics of the cornea in keratoconus and how it is altered in both geometrical and corneal material that should be accounted in order to have reliable and predictable results in ICRS surgery.

Chapter 6 describes biomechanical modeling of tonometry in order to have a better prediction of intraocular pressure measurements, accounting geometrical and material corneal parameters like thickness, Young's modulus, and curvature.

References

1. G.O. Waring, Making sense of keratospeak a classification of refractive corneal surgery. Arch. Ophthalmol. **103**(10), 1472–77 (1985)
2. R.L. Lindstrom, Minimally invasive radial keratotomy: mini-rk. J. Cataract Refract. Surg. **21** (1), 27–34 (1995)
3. A. Arciniegas, L.E. Amaya, Asociación de la queratotomía radial y la circular para la corrección de ametropías. Enfoque biomecánico, chapter XXII. Soc. Am. de Oftalmología, Bogotá (1981)
4. R.A. Villaseñor, G.R. Stimac, Clinical results and complications of trapezoidal keratotomy. J. Refract. Surg. **4**, 125–131 (1988)
5. Board of Directors of the International Society of Refractive Keratoplasty, Statement on radial keratotomy in 1988. J. Refract. Surg. **4**, 80–90 (1988)
6. M.J. Lynn, G.O. Waring III, R.D. Sperduto, The PERK Study Group, Factors affecting outcome and predictability of radial keratotomy in the perk study. Arch. Ophthalmol. **105**, 42–51 (1987)
7. K.A. Buzard, Introduction to biomechanics of the cornea. Refract. Corneal Surg. **8**(2), 127–138 (1992)
8. P.S. Binder, S.K. Nayak, J.K. Deg, E.Y. Zavala, J. Sugar, An ultrastructural and histochemical study of long-term wound healing after radial keratotomy. Am. J. Ophthalmol. **103**, 432–440 (1987)
9. G. Waring, S. Hannush, S. Bogan, R. Maloney, Classification of Corneal Topography with Videokeratography, in *Corneal Topography: Measuring and Modifying the Cornea*, ed. by D.J. Schanzlin, J. Robin (Springer, New York, 1992), pp. 70–71
10. J.Ø. Hjortdal, Regional elastic performance of the human cornea. J. Biomech. **29**, 931–942 (1996)
11. K.A. Buzard, B.R. Fundingsland, Assessment of corneal wound healing by interactive topography. J. Refract. Surg. **14**, 53–60 (1998)
12. Y.C. Fung, *Biomechanics: Mechanical Properties of Living Tissues* (Springer, New York, 1993)
13. P. Vena, R. Contro, Design sensitivity analysis of microdamage models for orthopaedic implants, in *CDROM Proc. Fourth World Congress on Comp. Mech.* (1998)
14. E. Di Martino, R. Pietrabissa, S. Mantero, The computational approach applied to the design and structural verification of a trileaflet polymeric heart valve. Adv. Eng. Softw. **28**, 341–346 (1997)
15. C.A. Taylor, G. Engel, T.J.R. Hughes, Finite element simulation of pulsatile flow through distensible blood vessels, in *CDROM Proc. Fourth World Congress on Comp. Mech.* (1998)
16. H.C. Howland, R.H. Rand, S.R. Lubkin, A thin-shell model of the cornea and its application to corneal surgery. Refract. Corneal Surg. **8**(2), 183–186 (1992)

Chapter 2
Corneal Biomechanics

Fabio A. Guarnieri

1 Introduction

The cornea is the first and most powerful refractive surface of the optical system of the eye.

The production of an accurate image in the retinal receptors requires the cornea to be transparent and have a suitable refractive power [1–3].

The structural integrity of the cornea can be altered in the CR modifying its refractive properties. These procedures have been developed empirically without detailed knowledge of corneal behavior.

Measuring the change in corneal shape has been available in the past decade through computerized analysis of the reflection of photokeratoscopic ring surface of the cornea (corneal topographer).

Little is known about the behavior of the internal structure of the cornea. Although the ultrastructure was analyzed by electron microscopy, the role of each one of the layers has not been examined in detail. We shall see below attempts to define such roles, which still need further analysis.

The tools to measure and understand these processes arise from mechanical engineering and have been used in other medical specialties, such as orthopedics, which evaluates quantitatively the requirements of the prosthesis. Many of these methods are not suitable for soft tissue such as the cornea, but the general principles can be applied.

F.A. Guarnieri, Ph.D. (✉)
Department of Bioengineering, Centro de Investigación de Métodos
Computacionales (CIMEC), Predio CONICET-Santa Fe, Colectora Ruta Nac 168,
Km 472, Paraje El Pozo, 3000 Santa Fe, Argentina
e-mail: aguarni@santafe-conicet.gov.ar

© Springer Science+Business Media New York 2015
F.A. Guarnieri (ed.), *Corneal Biomechanics and Refractive Surgery*,
DOI 10.1007/978-1-4939-1767-9_2

2   The Cornea

2.1   *Anatomical and Physical Properties*

The refractive power of the cornea depends on the curvature at its anterior and posterior surfaces, its thickness, and the refractive index difference between the air and the aqueous humor. The radius of curvature on the anterior surface of the cornea varies from the center (apex) toward the periphery. It is steeper in the central and somewhat flattened at the periphery. Average values of 7.8 and 6.7 mm from anterior to the posterior surface (Fig. 2.1).

At the apex, a wide range of variation of the radius of curvature of 7–8.5 mm is compatible with good visual function, and in pathological conditions increases even more the spectrum. Short radii result in refractive power and high myopia. Conversely, large rays give a low dioptric power and farsightedness. Furthermore, the central corneal curvature is often not equal in all meridians. The focus of the rays reflected by a point object does not form a point image on the retina. In these cases occurs astigmatism (a, without; stigma, point).

The curvature of the cornea changes somewhat with age. It is more spherical in childhood and changes to the rule astigmatism (more curved horizontal meridian) in adolescence.

Then again it becomes more spherical in adulthood to turn against the rule astigmatism (steepest vertical meridian) with senility.

The thickness also varies from the center to the periphery. This causes the difference in curvatures of the anterior and posterior surfaces. It has an average value of 0.5 mm center, increasing toward the periphery at an average of 1.2 mm at the limbus (limit of the cornea with sclera).

The corneal thickness is determined largely by corneal hydration that increases with increasing hydration and slightly with the age. The refractive index of the cornea is 1.376, and an average refractive power is 48.8 D (diopter). The concave posterior surface of the cornea is wetted by the aqueous humor, which has a lower refractive index (1.336), so that the average dioptric power in this area is −5.8 D.

To calculate the total dioptric power we rely on Gullstrand corneal thick lens equation, giving a value of 43 D, about 70 % of the overall refractive power of the eye. The lens only contributes 20 D convergence.

The cornea presents diurnal fluctuations in its topography in spite of relatively stable visual acuity. The factors involved in these variations are both physiological and anatomical, as the pressure of the eyelid, the time of day (especially during sleep), the tonicity of the tear film, and hormone levels.

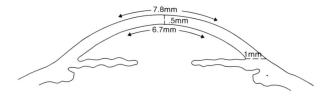

Fig. 2.1   Mean corneal radii
of curvature and thicknesses

Fig. 2.2 Scanning electron microscopy of ablated cornea with a 211-nm laser (picosecond). Magnification 550x (Xin-Hua Hu, Ph.D., UC Irvine, CA, EEUU)

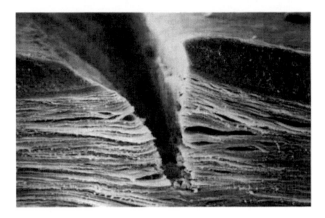

2.2   Histology of the Cornea

To perform a structural study of the cornea it is necessary to know not only the geometry but profoundly its internal components and functions performed to maintain corneal integrity. Furthermore, due to cuts or laser ablations performed in refractive surgery, it is vital to understand the healing process of wounds and scarring and to predict the refractive outcome of such processes. In Fig. 2.2, there is a scanning electron micrograph of an incision with laser wavelength of 211 nm, where the Bowman is observed (top) and multiple layers of collagen fibers.

The cornea is composed of five layers:

1. The epithelium consists of 5 or 6 layers of cells. The more superficial are flat and are superimposed like the skin, but are not keratinized. The following layers are arranged more stacked tightly together. Between epithelium and Bowman's membrane there is a basal membrane of 60–65 nm thick.
2. Epithelial cells form a layer of uniform thickness and great regularity. Their function is to maintain the stability of the tear film.
3. Bowman's membrane tissue is a transparent sheet of approximately 12 μm. It is acellular and is composed of densely packed collagen fibrils that are in random direction. Its absence in inferior animals is associated with a plasticity of corneal stroma.
4. The stroma is composed of film layers that run the entire length of the cornea; although the bundles are interlaced with each other, they are nearly parallel to the surface. The sheets are bonded together only loosely and are formed by bundles of collagen fibrils (bands of 64 nm) separated by a basic substance and water mucopolysaccharides. The latter are responsible for maintaining the hydration and transparency of the cornea and sclera that is not clear and does not contain mucopolysaccharides. The content of cells per unit volume is small. The cell bodies are flat, so they are also arranged parallel to the corneal surface. This arrangement of optical fibers provides uniformity to the cornea. The stroma constitutes approximately 90 % of the thickness of the cornea.

5. The Descemet membrane is approximately 10 nm thick. It is considered a secretion of endothelial cells. The membrane is comprised of type IV collagen fibers with similar characteristics to those of other basal membranes of blood vessels and lens capsule. It has a similar structure to the corneal stroma in terms of its regularity. It is highly elastic and represents a barrier against punctures.

The endothelium is a single layer of cells lining the Descemet membrane. Its inner surface is bathed by the aqueous humor. In humans the reproducibility of these cells is limited. The age causes cell loss and the remaining cells become larger and spread. Endothelial cells provide a barrier to the passage of water of the aqueous stroma. It prevents the cornea becoming hydrated with the aqueous humor. Cell losses are key factors the corneal edema and thickening of the thickness.

2.3   Corneal Wound Healing

The accidental or surgical injury of one or all of the layers of the cornea results in increased hydration and loss of transparency. Therefore, it is necessary and appropriate rapid healing of wounds to prevent scarring or opacities. The speed and the type of healing depend on several factors; among them are the anatomical location (limbal or corneal), the size of the wound, the layer of the cornea involved, bacterial, viral, or fungal infection, and drug administration therapeutic purposes. Thus, the damage of the corneal epithelium in general trauma heals in 24–48 h in a normal eye. Bacterial, viral, or fungal ulcers or those involving the deeper layers of the stroma can take weeks to heal. Therefore, deep laceration or surgical incision takes several weeks to heal completely.

The normal healing process of cuts on the central area of the cornea involves a cytological response and sleeve. Sometimes, for reasons not very clear, blood vessels can grow from the healed corneal tissue. The normal cornea is completely devoid of blood vessels. The capillaries extend just 1–2 mm beyond the limbal zone.

3   Measurements of the Mechanical Parameters

3.1   Extensibility of the Cornea

In 1937, Friedenwald [4] developed a formula which relates changes in intraocular pressure (IOP) with intraocular volume during Schiotz tonometry:

$$\log\frac{P}{P_0} = K\Delta V \tag{2.1}$$

where P_0 = initial pressure; P = pressure following the change of volume ΔV; K = coefficient of ocular rigidity.

Friedenwald established that the value of K eyes remained constant for pressure higher than 5 mmHg (133 Pa/mmHg).

Many researchers, including Gloster and Perkins in 1957, attempted to determine experimentally the rigidity coefficient. Contradictory results were obtained concluding that K is not constant in the physiological range of IOP.

Therefore, the formula (Eq. 2.1) was invalidated. It was suggested that studies of the extensibility of the cornea and sclera in uniaxial test could help explain such changes. Already in 1864, Schelske gave way to a coefficient of elasticity for the cornea and sclera of humans and rabbits. He found that the coefficient for meridional scleral strips was 7 % more extensible than the equatorial, and the cornea was twice extensible than sclera. Weber in 1877 had found a large variation in scleral extensibility strips between different human eyes. Perkins and Gloster performed extensibility measurements with corneal and scleral strips isolated from rabbits, using weights that produce stresses as close as possible to those of a normal eye. They compared these results with the determinations made by the authors of the intact eye strain. They found that the eye became less distensible at high pressures, consistent with the fact that the scleral strips became less extensible to the increased tension to a certain point (20 N/m) where extensibility became more constant. But they also noted that the strips did not return to their original length after the weights were removed. They found the creep phenomenon (temporary slow deformation with time) in strips with an instant length change of 81.8 % and 6' to reach the stationary state. During distension of the intact eye, the cornea and sclera extend in two directions where the stresses are distributed and the thickness decreases. In the case of uniaxial test strips there is a single direction, length, and decrease in both the thickness and width. Therefore, Perkins and Gloster did not justify performing a close analogy between distension of an intact eye and scleral and corneal strips.

Woo and Kobayashi [5] came to the same conclusion as Gloster and Perkins in human eyes. They added that exposing the free ends of collagen fibers caused a minor elastic response of the material and the straightening of the curved strips into a uniaxial test caused a significant error in elasticity measurements. They argued that it is important to consider, for volume changes to changes in IOP, the geometry variations and corneal material inhomogeneity. They did not consider the viscoelasticity and large deformations. Kobayashi and Woo devised a method for determining the elastic properties of the sclera and the cornea retaining its natural geometry. They sectioned equatorially enucleated eyes (1–3 days post mortem) and placed each half shell (anterior and posterior) in a pressure chamber. They found that both the shell and the subsequent previous corneosclera bear their weight without IOP. They measured with a scanner system the deformation of the horizontal surface while the pressure was increased. A photomultiplier detects the reflection of light at two targets located at two points of the cornea. The light was generated by a cathode ray tube driven by a triangular wave generator. They also measured lateral deformations (0°, 45°, 90°) to determine the isotropy of the material. They found that the deformation in three directions was very small. Moreover, they conducted a hysteresis test resulting in a minor viscoplastic (time dependent but not temporary deformation) effect. They considered the material as isotropic assuming that stresses across the thickness were only 10 % of the other planar strains in the corneal cap. Based on pressure–deformation curve measures, Woo and Kobayashi considered it also as nonlinear. In order to obtain stress–strain curves in the natural three-dimensional state of the cornea, they constructed a mathematical model [6] using effective stress and effective trilinear deformation.[1] The model parameters were adjusted iteratively until deformations predicted by finite element analysis agreed with those obtained experimentally (a technique called inverse method). Once the fit is reached, trilinear relations were converted to an exponential function through least squares method (best fit optimization method), obtaining

$$
\begin{aligned}
\sigma_e &= 18(e^{41.8\varepsilon_e} - 1)\text{kPa (stroma)} \\
\sigma_e &= 5.4(e^{28.0\varepsilon_e} - 1)\text{kPa (cornea)}
\end{aligned}
\tag{2.2}
$$

To validate the equation, a pressure–volume curve of the anterior segment of the eye was compared with experiments obtaining good agreement except for high pressure. Concentrated high stresses in clamped edges and possible swelling of the cornea by humid air are potentially the causes of high pressure discrepancy.

Schlegel et al. [7] investigated the viscoelastic properties in human enucleated eyes using ultrasonic waves by measuring changes in ocular diameter while IOP was cyclical. They found that pre-pressurized eyes had a substantially less viscoelastic response. Using the same protocol of Schlegel, Kobayashi et al. [8] determined the viscoelastic response of human corneas subjected to PIO from the same procedure of Woo et al. The purpose was to isolate the effect of viscoelastic pressure decay over time by measuring pressure with a tonometer. In pre-pressurized eyes the answer was almost negligible. The viscoelastic response was characterized in pre-pressurized eyes with a five-element linear viscoelastic model. They found average values of $53.68 \pm 83.03'$ to the slow time constant and $11.1 \pm 0.71'$ for the fast time constant. The average instantaneous elastic modulus was 1.11 MPa. A nonlinear viscoelastic mode l (Fung hereditary integral) found a better characterization of the viscoelastic parameters.

---

[1]

Effective stresses and strain are : $\sigma_e = \dfrac{1}{3}\sqrt{(\sigma_1 - \sigma_2)^2 + (\sigma_2 - \sigma_3)^2 + (\sigma_3 - \sigma_1)^2}$ and ε_e

$$
= \frac{2}{3}\sqrt{(\varepsilon_1 - \varepsilon_2)^2 + (\varepsilon_2 - \varepsilon_3)^2 + (\varepsilon_3 - \varepsilon_1)^2}
\tag{2.3}
$$

Greene and McMahon [9] studied in enucleated intact rabbit eyes the primary, secondary, and tertiary scleral creep function of temperature (26–48) and IOP (15–100 mmHg). In physiological conditions (37 °C and 15 mmHg), there is a speed creep of 0.06 %/h corresponding to 0.5 D/day. This measure has no physiological meaning in humans.

Russell and Klyce [10] modeled with FEM the corneal hydration regulation.

Parameters as permeability and solute transport through the intervening membrane were determined. It was simulated corneal hydration dynamics, thickness variations at different boundary conditions, such as hypertonic solutions, cold environments, high IOP (glaucoma), and destruction of limiting cell membranes (epithelium and endothelium). They predicted that the removal of the epithelium (as in laser photokeratectomy) causes an increase of the stromal thickness by 25 % for 1 h, consistent with the results in vivo.

Greene [11] examined the stresses undergone by posterior sclera at the accommodation produced by zonular fibers, convergence, vitreous pressure, and extraocular muscles. He noted that animals can myopize experimentally. He concluded that the oblique muscles are capable of originating local stress concentrations near the entry of the optic nerve.

Arciniegas et al. [12] found a relationship between the elastic modulus and the proportional limit with the age for high loads ($\sigma \gg 14$ kPa) in 24 eyes of 24 human scleras of various ages. They found that from birth both are high and decrease with age to stabilize after 20 years approximately. This reflects that the surgery should be performed after stabilization refraction. While there may be other parameters to ensure this, it is possible that there is a dependent refractive corneal elasticity. Creep was also measured in corneal-scleral shells of 30 rabbits being of 1.4222 %/h for 20 mmHg a value higher than in rabbits (Greene and McMahon). One important measurement in the diagnosis of glaucoma was to compare the pressure measurements with the Goldmann tonometer and a sensor implanted within the vitreous chamber of the eye of a rabbit. They found an average of 2.74 times greater IOP measurement with the sensor. Deficiencies the Goldmann tonometer is allotted not consider in corneal thickness, mechanical properties, the geometric shape of the eye, and creep.

Nash et al. [13] conducted a uniaxial test strips for low loads ($\sigma < 250$ kPa), finding the nonlinear relationship, but found no association with age eyes because they took ages over 20 years. They determined that the elasticity in normal corneas and keratoconus were equal. Creep was measured in human strips with a load of 150 psi for 2–20 h, finding similar results compared in Greene and McMahon.

Kamm and Battaglioli [14] found that the compressive Young's modulus through thickness is hundred times smaller than tensile (27–41 0.2 kPa). They also calculated Poisson's ratio across the thickness (0.46–0.50) resulting in a nearly incompressible material in that direction. However, they explained that the hydration and viscoelastic effect could influence the results, being even a lower compressive modulus.

3.2   Keratoconus Biomechanics

Edmund [15], in 1989, conducted a study of 27 patients with keratoconus and 37 normal to determine and describe corneal topography and pachymetry of their eyes and to evaluate the hypothesis that the difference is elastic. Methods and descriptive models were developed for characterizing corneal shape based on the central curvature and radial variation coefficient, eccentricity and function of the central curvature, the corneal thickness profile, fitted with a parabola, and the corneal-limbal ring, adjusted to an ellipse. Also, methods for estimating Young's modulus [16] and mass-based corneal topographic descriptive parameters were developed. An estimation of the stiffness from measurements of corneal tonometry with various weights and calibration tables from Friedenwald were derived.

He also showed that the stationary Young's modulus and stiffness (which would be related to instantaneous Young's modulus) is lower in keratoconus but have no correlation between them. It was shown that only in an advanced stage of keratoconus (>7.5 D) the corneal mass decreases. Based on the thickness and topographical changes, stress distribution is altered also based on the membranal theory (or law of Laplace) in keratoconic corneas. Tension along the meridian in normal corneas decreases while in keratoconic corneas increases. This increased tension would cause a second growth process of keratoconus in the corneal periphery as shown in the growth found in the periphery of the corneal thickness, contrary to the hypothesis of elastic keratoconus. It seems that the instantaneous Young's modulus reflects the immediate response of the collagen fibers, to match the value calculated from the ocular rigidity in comparison with the experimental measurements cornea strips. While the Young's modulus response appears to reflect steady elastic matrix glycosaminoglycans, consisting of the matrix compression and slippage of the collagen fibers, and that the estimated values are of the same order the Young's modulus of the matrix, also indicating that the collagen fibers are rather relaxed in the physiological state. This would be consistent with the theory that the slippage increases keratoconus collagen fibers due to reduced adhesion to Bowman's membrane and a matrix synthesis altered corresponding to an increase in the elasticity of the corneal tissue. Keratoconic biochemical studies demonstrating a normal collagen and altered proteoglycan synthesis confirm this hypothesis. On the influence of genetics and environment in keratoconus, see [Edmund] p. 30.

Hjortdal et al. [17] repeated the test of Woo and Kobayashi in ten corneas maintaining human corneal hydration normal IOP for a range of 2–10, 10–25, and 25–100 mmHg, finding values of 3, 9, and 20 MPa, respectively. The authors explain that the results of Woo and Kobayashi and Jue and Maurice give greater deformations due to greater corneal hydration. They assume that the values found still underestimate the Young's modulus values in a constant corneal volume.

In 1996, Hjortdal [18] studied in vitro the elasticity of the cornea and limbus by regions. He found rigidity at the limbus preferentially in a circumferential direction and to a lesser extent in the peripheral cornea preferentially in a meridional orientation. The same study was made after four radial keratotomy incisions by

Hjortdal et al. [19]. Normohydrated corneas were found to have an important role of local bending undamaged stromal tissue underneath the incision to generate the opening of the incision. He also found that compression of circumferential tissue disappears somewhere between the endothelium and epithelium to become taut.

Purslow et al. (1996) conducted a study of the relationship of IOP vs. volume based on the intrinsic stiffness Young's modulus. They found a relationship between the incremental values of Young's modulus at a given pressure proportion to the fourth power of the radius of the sphere eyepiece. They assumed that the Poisson's ratio is 0.5 confirming experimentally pachymetric measures.

3.3   Stromal and Descemet Membrane Extensibilities

Jue and Maurice [20] studied the mechanical properties of the stroma and Descemet membrane separately, using the principles of measuring the geometry of the intact eye.

The system consisted of a keratometer that viewed through a reflection prism two drops of mercury placed in the corneal surface. Full enucleated eyes were taken from rabbits and humans aged 45–90 years. Hysteresis tests were performed, responses to low and high tension, of the cornea intact isolated stromal and membrane isolation. Descemet's membrane is more extensible, in a nonlinear way. The stroma is virtually non-extensible and mimics intact corneal stromal mechanical properties.

From the high pressure curve, the elasticity modulus of the stroma is calculated. The stroma is composed of 70 % of its dry weight collagen fibers fi. The value of the elastic modulus of the collagen fibers can be obtained from the literature. Assuming constant voltage across the thickness, Laplace's equation gives the value for the case of spherical surfaces of thickness t radius of curvature R, under an internal pressure IOP

$$\sigma = \frac{P_{IO}R}{2t}; \quad \text{Laplace's equation} \tag{2.4}$$

Dry stromal thickness is 0.07 mm; therefore, the thickness of collagen in the stroma is equal to 0.05 mm. Curve obtained high pressures relationship IOP/e which is 9.106 Pa. Then within 7 mm, the Young's modulus ($E\,\sigma/\varepsilon$) of the stroma, without considering the extensibility of the ground substance, is in the order of 0.6 at 1 GPa. The procedure is to calculate the Young's modulus of Descemet's membrane at low tension. With a thickness of 12.5 µm, with a 150 cm H_2O/unidad deformation, Laplace equation leads to 5 MPa.

Considering the fundamental substance of stroma with a modulus of elasticity between 1 and 100 kPa (depending on stromal hydration) and as the volume ratio of collagen fibers and ground substance is 1:9 according to Maurice, we calculate the modulus of the stroma in fiber direction. This value has a range, depending on hydration of 11 MPa to 100 GPa.

Hanna et al. [21] used a mathematical technique to estimate the homogenization modulus of the stroma considering its fibrillar structure. This technique allows to describe macroscopic stress–strain relationship of materials whose microscopic structure is periodic. They conducted a model based on stromal microscopic measurements by X-ray diffraction of wet rat tendon similar (but not identical) to that of human corneal stroma and also based on transmission electron micrographs of human corneal stroma to estimate the relative contribution between the fibers and the ground substance. In the model we used the following values:

- Collagen fibers 35 % by volume
- Fiber diameter 25 nm
- Space between fibers 48 nm
- 20 % hydration fixed (both for fibers and for substance)
- E 1 GPa longitudinal fibers

Poisson's ratios calculated for the fibers and the ground substance and the Young's modulus for the basic substance, adjusting the coefficients until homogenization values, agreed with the experimental values found in the literature. The results are consistent with previous experiences, which validates the model clinically. For holographic interferometry, Kasprzak et al. [22] Elastic Modulus measured bovine corneal tangent for high pressures coincide with curves and Maurice Jue.

3.4 Bowman's Membrane Importance

There are controversies regarding the role of Bowman's membrane in corneal structure [23]. It is believed that Bowman's membrane contributes to the stability of the corneal curvature and is also protective against injury and infections. While it has not been shown experimentally, this hypothesis is taken into account in refractive surgery to preserve it.

On the contrary, in photorefractive keratectomy, made with UV excimer laser or IR, the flattening is achieved by removing tissue from the anterior surface of the cornea, sacrificing central portions of Bowman's membrane.

Clinical experiences indicate that Bowman's membrane should be incised for changes in the anterior corneal curvature in refractive procedures.

Incisions within the stroma without breaking the Bowman's membrane curvature will not change much anterior curvature, but it can change the posterior curvature. It is considered that the removal of part of the Bowman membrane Excimer laser is a potential source of instability in the cornea long term. Although such considerations have not been demonstrated clinically.

Theo Seiler et al. [24] conducted a study showing that after 6 months of an excimer laser photorefractive keratectomy, the refractive result was stable.

Hjortdal et al. [25] found no significant mechanical contribution of Bowman's membrane in the instantaneous or short-term response.

3.5 Viscoelastic Parameters

Theo Seiler et al. [24] conducted a study of the viscoelastic properties of strips of cornea without Bowman's membrane. Creep tests performed (tissue exposed to constant load, measuring the extent as a function of time) and stress relaxation (the tissue exposed to a constant elongation measuring the tension as a function of time) into strips enucleated eyes cornea. To remove the layer of Bowman, perform excimer laser keratectomy. The results showed that the strips of cornea are average stress–strain relationship with 5 % higher Bowman without it. This value could be higher because the experimental error was 10 %. Furthermore, viscoelastic properties in this experiment did not differ. They found a fast relaxation time of 10.58 and 269 s for the slow corneal stripping of Bowman's membrane.

Smolek et al. [26] obtained spectrum by applying shear compliance spectroscopy technique compliance dynamic mechanical cutting cylindrical specimens explanted human corneas, according to corneal hydration and temperature, and in the frequency range of 0.1 MHz–100 Hz found that a myopic cornea is significantly softer than emetrópicas corneas in both low and high frequencies. They found that thickness change varies with the shear compliance significantly (600 times of 0.2–1 mm at 1 Hz) and also corneal hydration and temperature change significantly the shear compliance. They considered that it is important to detect the frequency range interest 0.1 Hz–1 MHz

Buzard et al. [27] monitored every 1 min corneal topography after placing a Honan balloon for 5 min, increasing IOP to 30 mmHg. Normal corneas found that very little change topography after 3 min in contrast corneas after 3 months of radial keratotomy flattened almost 1 D to 0.40 D minute to 3 minute. At 9 months this group flattened 0.10 D per minute. On jobs investigating corneal hydration and its implications for the CR, we refer the reader to the references [28–30, 10].

4 Biomechanical Models

In 1972, Woo et al. [5] input the results of the characterization of corneal and scleral field into a mathematical model by EF human corneal-scleral shell. This model was used to compute the nonlinear relationship between the intraocular pressure (IOP) and the volume of the eye and analyze the structural response during applanation tonometry [31]. The model was axisymmetric, with the geometry based on an idealized eye quadrilaterals with 665528 nodes. Bowman's membrane had the same elastic properties with that of the stroma, Descemet's membrane, and the sclera. Poisson's ratio equal to 0.49 was considered. Tests were performed with Poisson's ratio of 0.5 obtained differences in voltages 0.5 % to an IOP of 17 mmHg. The limbus was modeled by varying the elastic modulus in seven increments between stromal and scleral modules. They found that the tensions were greater at the limbus and at the Ecuador than in other areas. Other studies found that the stiffness coefficient decreased when Friedenwald increased IOP. The results were similar to data obtained in vivo by several researchers, but differed from results obtained in enucleated eyes because the model did not consider the additional stiffness post mortem produced in the choroid. In the simulation of applanation, modified stroma elastic properties (modulus perpendicular to the plane of the cornea = 20 kPa) to account for the collapsing of the collagen fibers under compression tonometer indenter. In this area the bending rigidity is decreased. They found that it is consistent with empirical results.

In 1988, Hanna et al. [32] used the FEM to build a mathematical model of the eye that analyzes the stress–strain relationship of corneal-scleral shell. They used an axisymmetric model, without considering the curvature aspheric anterior cornea. Simulated lamellar keratectomy and laser myopic keratomileusis. The material used was linear, elastic, isotropic, and having a modulus of elasticity $E = 5$ MPa and $\nu = 0.49$. They did not consider the initial stress state. The mesh elements 600 comprising half with four elements in thickness. The results presented were stress curves, meridional circumferential compression and shear.

Membrane behavior found in the posterior half of the eye, from limbo, to match the thickness meridional and circumferential stresses (in-plane stresses). In the cornea they found a linear variation in the thickness of meridional and circumferential stresses. The stresses in the outer layers were lower than in the internal. At the limbus, they were reversed.

Compressive stresses were small void in the outer layer (relative to atmospheric) and equal to the IOP except around the eye at the limbus, where they found no explanation of fluctuation. The shear stresses were zero except at the limbus, where bending. Decreasing the thickness keratectomy, stress increases and the remainder meridional not altered. In keratomileusis, the central zone behaves like a membrane and the rest of the eye is not altered.

In 1989, Hanna et al. [33] created a mathematical model EF to simulate radial keratotomy. Corneal asphericity was considered by using Lotmar equation for the cornea, assuming a moderately myopic cornea (5–6 D). Corneal material was elastic, nonlinear, and isotropic. They used a Mooney–Rivlin model quasi-incompressible elasticity taking values of 2.2–2 MPa for cornea and sclera. They used a 2-layer 3D mesh with 27-node isoparametric elements. The incisions were not refined in the eye and considered axisymmetric considering a quarter mesh. Gullstrand optics was used to calculate the refractive changes. The stress distribution in a cornea without cuts was similar to earlier work except in the compressive stresses where values were different. Eight radial incisions showed the pattern of changes in meridional stresses and circumferential compression along a meridian. The model predicted the central flattening and steepening in the medial periphery. They showed the effect of the number of incisions, IOP, the thickness of the incision, incision length, the central radius of curvature, and Young's modulus, consistent with clinical studies [34], except for the effect of IOP, which was greater, and incision the length of small diameter optical zone with no effect. The authors suggest a nonlinear viscoelastic anisotropic full eye 3D model, including muscle forces. They made no quantitative clinical validation of the model.

Kwitko et al. [35] used a digital videokeratoscope system to evaluate changes in corneal topography after strabismus surgery practiced on extraocular muscles of 36 eyes of rabbits. They compared the results with the simulation of surgery in control eyes. They found the importance of considering the stress state of the extraocular muscles on the sclera, affecting corneal topography, corroborated by clinical studies. The material model was linear, elastic, and isotropic, in an eye with axisymmetric geometry. The mesh included two elements in the thickness of the sclera and 4 in the thickness of the cornea, with two closure elements representing the Bowman and Descemet's membrane. The limbus was modeled with triangular elements. Muscles were modeled as nodal forces and orbital tissues that stabilize the balloon radial elastic elements on the back of the ocular globe. They predicted qualitatively corneal topographic change strabismus surgery.

Rand et al. [36] introduced a model for studying human corneal refractive changes of radial keratotomy, using a thin spherical shell model that is linear and elastic. They assume axisymmetry and isotropy. The surgery is simulated by changing the Young's modulus and the thickness at the position of the incisions. The model behaves purely membranal. The results are compared with other models in FE, agreeing in some features, such as the effect of IOP, depth of incisions, and irregular topography in the optical zone.

Pinsky and Datye [37, 38] proposed a thick membrane model. The RK incisions were simulated by introducing anisotropy and inhomogeneity in the membrane stiffness. Pinsky et al. assume that the cornea does not support bending and the cut fibers lose their ability to load stress due to low shear modulus of the matrix. They use a linear elastic material with moderate rotations (nonlinear geometric), with a high Young's modulus calculated by considering the microstructure of the corneal stroma as a composite of collagen fibers with a small area and a matrix. The cornea is allowed to rotate in the limbus, whereas the collagen fibers are more oriented circumferentially and offer great resistance against expansion due to high hoop stress therein. The results are compared with surgeons nomograms known as Arrowsmith, Deitz, and Sawelson. The Young's modulus is calibrated to approximately match the nomograms.

Buzard et al. [39] used a model to simulate axisymmetrically an FE inflating a human enucleated eye and measure the lateral displacement. The mesh had two elements in thickness. The model successfully match experimental data for pressures around physiologic, being very stiff at low pressures. In another study [40] they measured with a Baribeau microscope with a resolution of 1 μm, the opening of the surgical incision in a diagram of four radial incisions in enucleated human eye with a 3-mm optical zone, increasing IOP 25–100 mmHg. Using 26 biomechanical eye model membranal theory and considering the average values of corneal thickness and curvature determined the Young's modulus of 7.58 MPa. The maximum dispersion 25 mmHg was 50 μm at a distance of 3.5 mm from the apex.

Sawusch et al. [41] conducted a study of the opening of the incision comparing the results with a geometric model called "tissue addition" and a model in EF. The tissue addition model assumes that the opening of the incision is initially filled by epithelial and fibrous tissue. This model correlated well with human studies. The model consisted in a finite element mesh of a quarter of the eye assuming radial symmetry, two elements in the thickness of the sclera and limbus, four elements for the cornea, and shell elements representing the Bowman and Descemet's membranes. An isotropic linear elastic material assuming small displacements was considered. For four incisions with a 4-mm optic zone and a central curvature of 44 D, the EF model predicted central flattening 3.05 D and an opening in the middle area of 47 μm cut. For the same cornea, an intrastromal cut predicted no significant topographical changes. It also predicted the opening is greater at the periphery than near the corneal center, which was confirmed by histopathological studies. The tissue addition model predicted 3.10 D of flattening by using the incision gape calculated using the FE model and histopathological studies.

Vito et al. [42] examined different models of EF cornea comparing them to determine the relative importance of factors such as boundary conditions, thickness, and the number of corneal layers needed to adequately model it. They validated the model with corneal tonometry studies [6]. Shell model was dismissed due to high gradients of stresses in the thickness during an indentation, despite having a low thickness/radius of curvature ($t/R = 0.0625$) ratio. They also considered important to use models with large deformations. They modeled axisymmetric meshes with different boundary conditions with and without limbo. The material was considered isotropic linear elastic and quasi-incompressible. It was found that for the inflation of the cornea with IOP of 20 mmHg, the model with free boundary without limbo approached a membrane model. The same occurred in the central area of the model with free boundary in limbus and the horizontal direction. For the same model it was found that a higher elastic modulus of 2 MPa produced no changes in central curvature, showing a membrane behavior in the central area, and that the bending is only important in the contour. Different models with the membrane theory were compared with tonometry. Contact with the indenter using gap elements was also modeled.

It was shown to be necessary to consider geometric nonlinearity in the model. The boundary conditions did not affect the result. They introduced a model of corneal layers free to slide without friction between them. Their behavior, as the number of layers is increased, approached the membranal. The pressure distribution at the interface between the cornea and the indenter is not uniform. This indicates that the bending is important in tonometry, which would explain the discrepancies found between the tonometry and direct measurement of the IOP [43]. They also used this dependence to estimate the bending rigidity of the cornea [44].

Wray et al. [45] developed a 3D model of a fragment symmetrical to radial keratotomy eye including corneal nonlinear properties of the material obtained from in vivo data. Generally were selected as the constitutive equation proposed by Woo et al. [6]. Then they adjusted the parameters using in vivo data from a study of radial keratotomy in 290 eyes and performed a sensitivity study of different surgical parameters, obtaining comparable results with reality.

5 Toward a Computer-Aided Design of the Refractive Surgery

These papers consider the cornea as axisymmetric without cuts, i.e., the cornea is equivalent to a sphere. Thus, it is only possible to represent corneas with nearsightedness and farsightedness. It is possible to represent different cases of astigmatism (myopic, hyperopic, mixed). Neither is it possible to represent real corneas where the vertical diameter is less than the horizontal. Besides the geometrical data are obtained from the information keratometer, which only measures the average curvature of the corneal apex to 3 mm. It has been found that the error in systems based on corneal spherical mapping aspherical surfaces (such as the cornea after surgery) is significant [46].

Regarding the model of corneal material, nonlinearity has been modeled in small deformations by Woo et al. Bryant et al. attempted to adjust the experimental curves with hyperelastic models without result. No model represents the long-term effect of the cornea. There are attempts to model the effect of the corneal viscoelasticity Le Tallec [47, 48], but no clinical nor numerical data validation was found.

The author's thesis [49] developed a biomechanical model of the cornea incorporating the following guidelines:

- Precise geometric model incorporating technological advances in data acquisition such as corneal digital videokeratoscope and ultrasonic pachymetry [50, 51]
- Optical model suitable for further processing and suitable for clinical analysis ophthalmologist
- Suitable material model to mimic the behavior in the different corneal refractive surgery procedures, both in the short and long term
- Validation of elements with real patient data

This required the following characteristics of the model:

1. The 3D geometry, with change of corneal thickness, performing an interface with the data acquisition equipment
2. Optical thick lenses and topographic map to evaluate results
3. Hyperelastic nonlinearity viscoelastic material

April. Actual patient data (topography, pachymetry, clinical data, pre- and postsurgical) for radial and astigmatic keratotomy and excimer laser photokeratectomy

Figure 2.3 is a flow diagram to model the cornea.

Simulador cirugía ocular

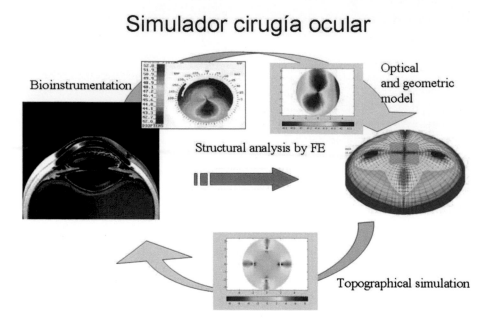

Fig. 2.3 Flow diagram to model the cornea

6 Data Acquisition

Optical and geometric data were obtained from instrumentation commonly used in the ophthalmology clinic (there is no instrumentation that obtains the spatial geometry of the cornea in a direct way). The ultrasonic pachymeter, a slit lamp, and a digital videokeratoscope were used.

6.1 Corneal Thickness

The ultrasonic pachymeter utilized point measurements performed on the cornea. It was assumed that the measurements were made normal to the anterior corneal surface. Initially two steps, one at the apex and another at the limbus (corneal periphery), were performed. Edmund [15] described a parabolic variation between the central thickness and the peripheral

$$T(x) = T\left(1 + T_V x^2\right) \tag{2.5}$$

where $T(x)$ is the corneal thickness on the chord segment x from the apex. T denotes the central corneal thickness. T_V is defined as the coefficient of variation of thickness and is constant.

6.2 Corneal-Limbal Ring

Corneal-limbal ring (CLR) denotes the boundary between the cornea and the remaining eye most highly curved.

Through a slit lamp it is possible to measure corneal diameters. Generally, the vertical to the horizontal diameter is less than 1 or about 2 mm. The CLR was adopted as an ellipse where a and b are the major and minor diameters of the ellipse:

$$y^2 = b^2 - \frac{b^2}{a^2} x^2 \tag{2.6}$$

where a and b are the diameters of the ellipse.

6.3 Anterior Surface

The corneal topographer (e.g., EyeSys) is based on equally spaced projecting concentric rings onto the cornea (Placido disk) where radius maps are obtained. They are deployed in one angular degree separated by meridians. The detailed description of the algorithm is in reference [52].

The rate of change of direction (curvature) at a point is (for flat curves)

$$\kappa = \frac{z_{,rr}}{\left(1 + z_{,r}^2\right)^{3/2}} = \frac{1}{\rho} \tag{2.7}$$

Assuming smoothness and the center of the cornea is the apex (condition alleged by the corneal topographer) is possible to calculate the elevation at each meridian. Differential equation is solved in each meridian z assuming a variation of the radius of curvature in one direction, the meridional. This hypothesis agrees with that made by the reconstruction algorithm of the corneal topographer.

The posterior surface is generated from the spatial coordinates of the anterior surface calculated and the thickness measured (typically 5,760 points).

6.4 Intraocular Pressure

The intraocular pressure (IOP) is measured with a Goldmann tonometer [31]. There are controversies on the validity of the ocular tonometry, especially for corneas that do not approach the average eye (thin corneas, very elastic, very rigid, very flat or highly curved, very aspherical) [3].

6.5   Ocular Length and Depth of the Anterior Chamber

A-scan ultrasonographer (linear 1D) measures the length of the eye, the depth of anterior chamber, and the axial crystalline lens axially from the cornea of the eye to the fovea. This length allows the full refraction of the eye and along with the corneal and lens refraction the calculus of the total refraction required to correct ametropia (Fig. 2.4).

Chamber depth is the distance between the cornea and iris. It is about a few millimeters. It can be measured with a B-mode ultrasound sensor (sweep 2D) (Fig. 2.5).

6.6   Objective and Subjective Refraction

Higher aberrations can be measured by Foucault knife-edge test, which retinoscopy is based, where a very small source is used to analyze aberrations of the eye. In order to quantify the wave aberration function, interferometry is being used in a modified Twyman–Green arrangement [53].

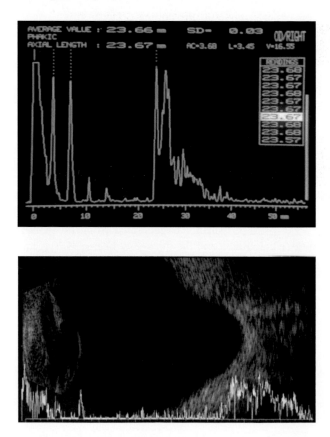

Fig. 2.4 A-scan
ultrasonographer

Fig. 2.5 B-mode
ultrasonography

7 Optical Model

It is important to determine the optical model of the eye in a biomechanical model that includes an analysis of stresses and strains. These strains will alter eye refraction.

In the author's thesis [49] a three-dimensional optical model was developed taking into account the optics of thick lenses. The diopter power of each of the components in the complete refractive eye (cornea, aqueous humor, lens, vitreous, and retina) considering a paraxial theory assumed by the disk-based corneal topography (Placido) and keratometry was calculated [54]. This allowed increase accuracy in evaluating the results of refractive surgery simulation so as the procedure performed on the actual patient.

It is also important in the optical model considering the number of points acquired and interpolated in corneal topography and pachymetry. This will allow to generate the geometry of the biomechanical model and the precision of the structural analysis of stresses and strains, which, as previously stated, will determine the precision of the optical analysis post biomechanical changes in eye structure. In the author's thesis [49] data for mesh generation needed in structural finite element analysis are prepared by an interpolation by moving-least-squares [55] allowing the use of different types of corneal topographers (based and not based on Placido disks).

In postprocessing the point-to-point curvature is calculated on the anterior surface carrying a map of diopters, which simulate the corneal topography. An ophthalmologist would compare preoperative and postoperative topography (simulated). An estimate of the dioptric power of the refractive system of the eye is performed after the simulation, analyzing the outcome of refractive surgery with the desired results.

7.1 Generation of Incisions

Radial keratotomy and arcuate keratotomy were simulated. It was necessary to perform a model of the incision that affects the geometry of the corneal structure. The characteristics of the relaxing incisions are:

- Depth variation.
- Incision with the scalpel does not remove tissue.
- Not create perforations (not touch Descemet's membrane).
- The incision space is completely filled with scar tissue.
- The incision is perpendicular to the corneal surface.

8 Mechanical Models

Finite elements based on elastic, hyperelastic, and viscoelastic theories were implemented. Both small and large displacements and deformations are taken into account.

8.1 Elastic Model

A linear isoparametric solid element with geometric nonlinearity and linear elastic and isotropic material was implemented. The values of Young's modulus and Poisson's constant were taken from [41, 56]. The corneal ortotropicidad was not initially considered because we assume that the stresses in the direction perpendicular to the corneal plane are negligible, compared to the stresses in that plane. These considerations were made following the work of Woo and Kobayashi [5].

8.2 Hyperelastic Model

In order to consider the nonlinearity materials described in the work of Woo and Kobayashi hyperelastic model was performed. The material models were implemented: (1) Blatz–Ko, for compressible hyperelastic; (2) Mooney–Rivlin, for quasi-incompressible; (3) Hart–Smith, for quasi-incompressible; (4) and a new exponential hyperelastic model developed in this thesis for human corneal tissue and other biological materials with high nonlinearity.

To adjust the models with experimental tests, tensile test on strips of cornea and inflation tests were used in intact eye. The new model was the only one capable of adjusting the intact cornea test in the inflated, i.e., beginning with IOP = 0, due to the highly nonlinear.

The materials in the test model of corneal inflation parameters, fitted using an axisymmetric model as a numerical optimization scheme via finite element method (inverse method). The parameters were varied in an iterative manner based on a nonlinear optimization algorithm originally implemented by R. Hooke and T.A. Jeeves [57]. The error function consisted of the mean square error between the experimental curve of corneal inflation and simulation analysis in FE.

8.3 Viscoelastic Model

To take into account the viscoelastic properties of the cornea and predict the response to medium term refractive surgery, finite element corneal model was performed using a 3-element model (Zener type) in large deformations. The viscoelastic parameters were adjusted to experimental creep and dynamic tests with sinusoidal load on corneal strips.

9 Boundary Conditions

Given that the model of the cornea is a part of the complete structure of the eye, special considerations must be taken when defining the boundary conditions. If the spherical eye was considered, taking only the cornea in the model, it would be enough, as boundary conditions, to restrict the movement toward the sclera or to the rest of the eye.

But the cornea is aspherical, and the radius of curvature of the sclera is not equal to the radius of curvature of the cornea. The limbus is the transition zone between these radii of curvature. From the spatial reconstruction of topographic data, it is not possible to determine the geometry of limbus since the corneal topographer does not measure its curvature.

Following the work of Datye and Pinsky [37, 38], the cornea is allowed to rotate, considering that the collagen fibers are oriented circumferentially to this area.

10 Initial Conditions

Corneal deformation under the effect of relaxing incisions in the refractive surgery is caused by the intraocular pressure. Assuming that the intraocular pressure is constant before and after the operation performed, the effect is attributed to the change in thickness located in the incised area, causing a change in the stress of the affected tissue and a deformation on the initial state.

11 Summary

A number of studies have been undertaken in an attempt to characterize the mechanical properties of the cornea. The corneal biomechanics has been described by in vitro simple tension [4, 12, 13, 24, 58], inflation [5, 17, 20, 56, 59], and compression tests [14]. The biomechanical response of the cornea *in surgical procedures* has been described mostly for radial keratotomy by measuring local deformations [19, 40, 60]. Others have used finite element models with different assumptions regarding corneal geometry and material properties. Some have assumed that the cornea is a homogeneous linear elastic [42, 52, 61], nonlinear elastic [21, 45, 56, 60] solid, and nonhomogeneous membrane [38].

Attempts to verify the models have been done with inlations tests [56] in hydrated corneas and with local deformations [60] in normo-hydrated corneas. The relationship between corneal strain and intraocular pressure was found to be nonlinear, showing a typical stress-stiffening behavior. A material model by Woo et al. [5] has been used to account that nonlinearity [45, 56, 60].

The anisotropy of the cornea is evidenced by its microstructure as a reinforced composite with collagen fibers immersed in a jelly-like matrix of mucopolysaccharides. There have been attempts to account the anisotropy of the cornea, with transverse isotropy, but since the cornea is also nearly incompressible [14] violates the restrictions on the elastic constants [62]. Pinsky et al. modeled the anisotropy produced by the relaxing incisions in a thick membrane model. But local bending effects near the incision were found to be an important factor [19].

The hydration has a profound effect on the extensibility of the stroma [19], and viscoelastic properties have been measured in vivo after radial keratotomy [27]. A complete model of the cornea should take into account the poroelasticity, viscoelasticity, and anisotropicity of the cornea.

Hyperelastic models are proper for material and geometrical nonlinearities. Geometric nonlinearities appear in inflation tests as well as in refractive procedures like those involving the insertion of intrastromal rings. They are also suitable for further extension to anisotropy and inelasticity. There were attempts to use rubber-based hyperelastic models, like Mooney–Rivlin [33, 56] and Ogden [56], but they did not reproduce the high nonlinearity of the cornea.

In the next chapters it will be described a hyperelastic model that accounts for the nonlinearity of the cornea, both material and geometrical, and is suitable for viscoelasticity [63] and poroelasticity. Inflations tests [56, 17, 62] in hydrated and normo-hydrated corneas will be used to obtain the material parameters of the model and simulate and attempt to predict the behavior of relaxing incisions, ablation of the cornea and insertion of intrastromal ring segments to correct different ametropias (myopia, hypermetropy, astigmatism) and keratoconus.

References

1. R. Moses, W. Hart(h), *Fisiologia del Ojo. Aplicacion clinica.* (Adler. Panamericana, Bs.As. 1988)
2. R. Berne, M. Levy, *Fisiologia.* (Panamericana, Bs. As., 1986)
3. D. Schanzlin, J. Robin, *Corneal Topography. Measuring and Modifying the Cornea* (Springer, New York, 1992)
4. J. Gloster, E.S. Perkins, M.-L. Pommier, Extensibility of strips of sclera and cornea. British. J. Ophthal. **41**, 103–110 (1957)
5. S.L.-Y. Woo, A.S. Kobayashi, W.A. Schlegel, C. Lawrence, Nonlinear material properties of intact cornea and sclera. Exp. Eye Res. **14**, 29–39 (1972)
6. S.L.-Y. Woo, A.S. Kobayashi, W.A. Schlegel, C. Lawrence, Mathematical model of the corneo-scleral shell as applied to intraocular pressure–volume relations and applanation tonometry. Ann. Biomed. Eng. **1**, 87–89 (1972)

7. W.A. Schlegel, C. Lawrence, L.G. Staberg, Viscoelastic response in the enucleated human eye. Investigat. Ophthalmol. **11**(7), 593–599 (1972)

8. A.S. Kobayashi, L.G. Staberg, W.A. Schlegel, Viscoelastic properties of human cornea. Exp. Mech. **13**(12), 497–503 (1973)

9. P.R. Greene, T.A. McMahon, Scleral creep vs. temperature and pressure in vitro. Exp. Eye Res. **29**, 527–537 (1979)

10. S.D. Klyce, S.R. Russell, Numerical solution of coupled transport equations applied to corneal hydration dynamics. J. Physiol. **292**, 107–134 (1979)

11. P.R. Greene, Mechanical considerations in myopia: relative effects of accommodation, convergence, intraocular pressure and the extraocular muscles. Am. J. Optom. Physiol. Opt. **57**, 902–914 (1980)

12. A. Arciniegas, L.E. Amaya, Asociacion de la *queratotomia radialy la circular para la correccion de ametropias. Enfoque biomecdnico,* chapter XXII. Soc. Am. de Oftalmologi'a, Bogota, (1981)

13. I.S. Nash, P.R. Greene, C.S. Foster, Comparison of mechanical properties of keratoconus and normal corneas. Exp. Eye Res. **35**, 413–423 (1982)

14. J.L. Battaglioli, R.D. Kamm, Measurements of the compressive properties of scleral tissue. Invest. Ophthalmol. Vis. Sci. **114**(2), 202–215 (1992)

15. C. Edmund, Corneal topography and elasticity in normal and keratoconic eyes. Acta Ophthalmol. **193**, 1–36 (1989)

16. E. Sjontoft, C. Edmund, In vivo determination of young's modulus for the human cornea. Bull. Math. Biol. **49**, 217–232 (1987)

17. J.O. Hjortdal, N. Ehlers, Extensibility of the normo-hydrated human cornea. Acta Ophthalmol. Scand. **73**(1), 12–17 (1995)

18. J.O. Hjortdal, Regional elastic performance of the human cornea. J. Biomech. **29**, 931–942 (1996)

19. J.O. Hjortdal, N. Ehlers, Acute tissue deformation of the human cornea after radial keratotomy. J. Refract. Surg. **12**(3), 391–400 (1996)

20. B. Jue, D. Maurice, The mechanical properties of the rabbit and human cornea. J. Biomech. **19** (10), 847–854 (1986)

21. K.D. Hanna, F.E. Jouve, G.O. Waring III, Computer simulation of arcuate keratotomy for astigmatism. Refract. Corneal Surg. **8**(2), 152–163 (1992)

22. H. Kasprzak, W.N. Forster, G. von Bally, Measurement of elastic modulus of the bovine cornea by means of holographic interferometry. Part 1. Method and experiment. Optom. Vis. Sci. **70**(7), 535–544 (1993)

23. E. Yavitz, Reshaping the cornea. Ocular Surg. News, Online article, p. 3, April 1996

24. T. Seiler, M. Matallana, S. Sendler, T. Bende, Does Bowman's layer determine the biomechanical properties of the cornea? Refract. Corneal Surg. **8**(2), 139–142 (1992)

25. J.O. Hjortdal, N. Ehlers, Effect of excimer laser keratectomy on the mechanical performance of the human cornea. Acta Ophthalmol. Scand. **73**(1), 18–24 (1995)

26. F. Soergel, B. Jean, T. Seiler, T. Bende, S. Miicke, W. Pechhold, L. Pels, Dynamic mechanical spectroscopy of the cornea for measurement of its viscoelastic properties in vitro. German J. Ophthalmol. **4**, 151–156 (1995)

27. K.A. Buzard, B.R. Fundingsland, Assessment of corneal wound healing by interactive topography. J. Refract. Surg. **14**, 53–60 (1998)

28. G. Simon, Q. Ren, Biomechanical behavior of the cornea and its response to radial keratotomy. Refract. Corneal Surg. **10**(3), 343–356 (1994). Comments by R. K. Maloney, S. T. Feldman and K. Buzard

29. P. Roy, W.M. Petroll, A.E. McKinney, C.J. Chuong, Computational models of the effects of hydration on corneal biomechanics and the results of radial keratotomy. J. Biomech. Eng. **118**, 255–258 (1996)

30. M.R. Bryant, P.J. McDonnell, A triphasic analysis of corneal swelling and hydration control. J. Biomech. Eng. **120**(3), 370–381 (1998)

31. H. Goldmann, Applanation tonometry, in *Glau-coma,* ed. by F.W. Newell, Trans. 2nd. Conference, Josiah Macy, Jr. Foundation, N. Jersey, 1959, pp. 167–220
32. K.D. Hanna, F.E. Jouve, M.H. Bercovier, G.O. Waring III, Computer simulation of lamellar keratectomy and laser myopic keratomileusis. Refract. Corneal. Surg. **4**, 222–231 (1988)
33. K.D. Hanna, F.E. Jouve, G.O. Waring III, Preliminary computer simulation of the effects of radial keratotomy. Arch. Ophthalmol. **107**, 911–918 (1989)
34. M.J. Lynn, G.O. Waring III, R.D. Sperduto, The PERK Study Group, Factors affecting outcome and predictability of radial keratotomy in the perk study. Arch Ophthalmol. **105**, 42–51 (1987)
35. S. Kwitko, M.R. Sawusch, P.J. McDonnell, H. Moreira, D.C. Gritz, D. Evensen, Efecto de la cirugi'a de los musculos extraoculares sobre la topografi'a corneal. Arch. Ophthalmol. (ed. esp.) **2**(6), 68–73 (1991)
36. R.H. Rand, S.R. Lubkin, H.C. Howland, Analytical model of corneal surgery. J. Biomech. Eng. **113**(2), 239–241 (1991)
37. P.M. Pinsky, D.V. Datye, A microstructurally-based finite element model of the incised human cornea. J. Biomech. **24**(10), 907–922 (1991)
38. P.M. Pinsky, D.V. Datye, Numerical modeling of radial, astigmatic and hexagonal keratotomy. Refract. Corneal Surg. **8**(2), 164–172 (1992)
39. K.A. Buzard, Introduction to biomechanics of the cornea. Refract. Corneal Surg. **8**(2), 127–138 (1992)
40. K.A. Buzard, J.F. Ronk, M.H. Friedlander, D.J. Tepper, D.A. Hoeltzel, K. Choe, Quantitative measurement of wound spreading in radial keratotomy. Refract. Corneal Surg. **8**(3), 217–223 (1992)
41. M.R. Sawusch, P.J. McDonnell, Computer modeling of wound gape following radial keratotomy. Refract. Corneal Surg. **8**(2), 143–145 (1992)
42. R.P. Vito, P.H. Carnell, Finite element method based mechanical models of the cornea for pressure and indenter loading. Refract. Corneal Surg. **8**(2), 146–151 (1992)
43. A. Arciniegas, L.E. Amaya, L.M. Hernandez, Physical factors that influence the measurement of the intraocular pressure with Goldmann's tonometer. New Trends Ophthalmol. **1**(1), 170–200 (1986)
44. P.H. Carnell, R.P. Vito, A model for estimating corneal stiffness using an indenter. J. Biomech. Eng. **114**(4), 549–552 (1992)
45. W.O. Wray, E.D. Best, L.Y. Cheng, A mechanical model for radial keratotomy: toward a predictive capability. J. Biomech. Eng. **116**(1), 56–61 (1994)
46. C. Roberts, Characterization of the inherent error in a spherically-biased corneal topography system in mapping a radially aspheric surface. Refract. Corneal Surg. **10**, 103–111 (1994)
47. P. Le Tallec, C. Rahier, A. Kaiss, Three-dimensional incompressible viscoelasticity in large strains: Formulation and numerical approximation. Comput. Methods Appl. Mech. Eng. **109**, 233–258 (1993)
48. P. Le Tallec, C. Rahier, Numerical models of steady rolling for non-linear viscoelastic structures in finite deformations. Int. J. Numer. Methods Eng. **37**, 1159–1186 (1994)
49. F.A. Guarnieri, Modelo Biomecanico del Ojo para Diseno Asistido por Computadora de la Cirugia Refractiva. PhD Dissertation, FICH-INTEC, Universidad Nacional del Litoral, Santa Fe, Argentina, 1999
50. F.A. Guarnieri, A. Cardona, Computer simulation of refractive surgery by using a finite element model, in *Abstract in Proceedings World Congress on Medical Physics and Biomedical Engineering, Rio de Janeiro, Brazil,* 1994
51. F.A. Guarnieri, A. Cardona, Videokeratoscope-based computer simulation of the refractive surgery. IEEE Trans. Biomed. Eng. (1998). Report to CONICET
52. F.A. Guarnieri, Modelo biomecanico del ojo para diseno asistido por computadora de la cirugi'a refractiva. Proyecto de grado de bioingeniena, Facultad de Ingeniena, UNER, Oro Verde, Entre Ri'os, Argentina, 1993

53. G. Smith, *The Eye and Visual Optical Instruments* (Cambridge University Press, New York, 1997)
54. D.B. Henson, *Optometric Instrumentation*, 2nd edn. (Butterworth-Heinemann, Oxford, 1996)
55. F.A. Guarnieri, A. Cardona, Moving least square method in the simulation of the corneal topography by fe in the refractive surgery, in *Congreso Argentino de Mecanica Computacional (ENIEF 95), Bariloche, Argentina*, 1995
56. M.R. Bryant, P.J. McDonnell, Constitutive laws for biomechanical modeling of refractive surgery. J. Biomech. Eng. **118**, 473–481 (1996)
57. M.G. Johnson, Nonlinear Optimization using the algorithm of Hooke and Jeeves, 1994. Documentacion en codigo fuente en C.
58. D.A. Hoeltzel, P. Altman, K.A. Buzard, K. Choe, Strip extensiometry for comparison of the mechanical response of bovine, rabbit and human corneas. J. Biomech. Eng. **114**(2), 202–215 (1992)
59. A. Nevyas-Wallace, Pattern recognition in subclinical and clinical keratoconus using elevation-based topography, in *Abstracts in Pre-AAO. ISRS*, 1996, p. 98
60. W.M. Petroll, P. Roy, C.J. Chuong, B. Hall, H.D. Cavanagh, J.V. Jester, Measurement of surgically induced corneal deformations using three-dimensional confocal microscopy. Cornea **15**(2), 154–164 (1996)
61. S.C. Velinsky, M.R. Bryant, On the computer-aided and optimal design of keratorefractive surgery. Refract. Corneal Surg. **8**(2), 173–182 (1992)
62. M. Sutcu, Orthotropic and transversely isotropic stress-strain relations with built-in coordinate transformations. Int. J. Solids Struct. **29**(4), 503–518 (1992)
63. F.A. Guarnieri, A. Cardona, 3d viscoelastic nonlinear incompressible finite element in large strain of the cornea. application in refractive surgery. in *Articles in CD-ROM Fourth World Congress of Computational Mechanics*, 1998

Chapter 3
Biomechanics of Incisional Surgery

Fabio A. Guarnieri

1 Introduction

Cornea is the main responsible of the refraction of the eye. Its structural properties are changed in Refractive Surgery [1], a technique used in ophthalmology to modify the refractive properties of the optical system of the eye. It is used in the correction of several ametropias like myopia, astigmatism, and hypermetropia. Among the different procedures, radial keratotomy, photorefractive keratectomy, and keratomileusis are commonly used in clinical practice. Radial keratotomy [2] is based on diamond knife relaxing incisions along the cornea, with maximum depth, but without perforation. The refractive change is reached by means of the action of the intraocular pressure over the relaxed cornea, by steepening where the thickness is smaller (at the incisions) and by flattening the uncut central zone to correct myopia 1 (Fig. 1.1).

The calculation of the incisions is undertaken commonly by means of nomograms or tables from previous experience. Some techniques involve the use of closed equations based on simple models. These techniques can leave the patient with significant overcorrection and undercorrection [3–6] since they do not contemplate the complexity of the cornea (irregular topography, anisotropy, viscoelasticity, etc.) nor the overall structure (sclera, ocular muscles, optical nerve and eyelids effects, etc.).

Mechanical engineering principles may be used to obtain a mathematical model of the cornea and provide help in the study of the corneal biomechanics, as well as predict its behavior.

F.A. Guarnieri, Ph.D. (✉)
Department of Bioengineering, Centro de Investigación de Métodos
Computacionales (CIMEC), Predio CONICET-Santa Fe, Colectora Ruta Nac 168,
Km 472, Paraje El Pozo, 3000 Santa Fe, Argentina
e-mail: aguarni@santafe-conicet.gov.ar

© Springer Science+Business Media New York 2015   33
F.A. Guarnieri (ed.), *Corneal Biomechanics and Refractive Surgery*,
DOI 10.1007/978-1-4939-1767-9_3

The cornea can be considered as a structure under pressure loading (atmospheric in the anterior surface, intraocular in the posterior surface), attached to a different structure as the sclera. By obtaining the structural material parameters (Young's modulus, Poisson's ratio, etc.), the actuating force values (intraocular pressure, lids effects, etc.), and the geometry (thicknesses and topography), it is possible to develop a structural analysis based on the finite element method [7].

The radial incisions of radial keratotomy can be simulated by modifying the geometry of the intact cornea. Thus the intraocular pressure actuates over the incised cornea and changes its curvature. The new geometry is stored and processed to determine the optical effects and verify the surgical planning proposed by the ophthalmologist.

2 Geometry from Corneal Topography

Patient data were obtained from medical instrumentation commonly used in ophthalmology. The intraocular pressure was measured with an applanation tonometer [8], the corneal thicknesses with a digital pachymeter [9], and a map of curvature radii with a digital videokeratoscope (corneal topographer) [10]. Figure 3.1 shows topographical color map of the curvature, measured in diopters (D) from a patient cornea.

The corneal structural parameters are difficult to measure in vivo. Several authors [11–16] present values for the Young's modulus and the Poisson's ratio for some layers of the cornea and sclera.

In order to introduce the corneal geometry of each patient, we developed an interface with the corneal topographer and a preprocessing stage to reconstruct the spatial geometry from curvature data. The considered criterion to determine

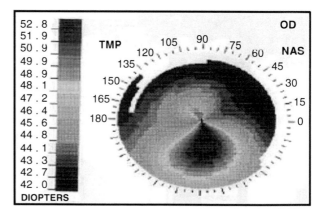

Fig. 3.1 The dioptric plot is color-coded so that steep and flat areas on the cornea can be easily visualized. An eye with irregular astigmatism is shown

the error in the reconstruction was the corneal topographer resolution (± 0.25 D). The elevation z *was* obtained in each meridian by solving the differential equation

$$\kappa = \frac{z_{,rr}}{\left(1 + z_{,r}^2\right)^{3/2}} = \frac{1}{\rho} \tag{3.1}$$

where $z_{,r}$ and $z_{,rr}$ are the first and second derivatives in radial direction.

This interface with the corneal topographer has the advantage to allow reconstructing the corneal geometry in each patient without any geometrical simplification (as the sphere–cylindrical corneal shape assumption). Previous works used this assumption [14–20]. Moreover, both central and peripheral refractions are considered.

3 Finite Element Analysis

A structured four-layer mesh with isoparametric solid elements was considered. Linear interpolation and linear elastic and isotropic material are used to represent the cornea. Transverse isotropy was neglected, since we assume stresses in the perpendicular direction to the corneal plane are negligible when compared with stresses in the corneal plane. These assumptions were stated by following the Woo and Kobayashi studies [12].

In order to set the material properties of the cornea, different authors, as seen in Chap. 2 [11–16], present values for Young's modulus and Poisson constant for the stroma and sclera. In a preliminary work values like 3 MPa and 0.48 were introduced in a finite element model, respectively.

Since the corneal model involves a portion of the eye, it is necessary to take special considerations in the boundary conditions of the model [18]. Since collagen fibrils at the limbus are oriented circumferentially (whereas they are oriented randomly in the cornea), we have considered the cornea to be hinged at the limbus as a boundary condition.

We inflate the unincised and incised models and subtract the curvature between them to obtain the final result. This procedure was compared successfully with other methods that disinflate iteratively the unincised model to obtain the initial unpressurized model.

3.1 Generation of the Incision

Incisions with diamond knife do not remove tissue and should not perforate the cornea, keeping the Descemet's layer intact. The gape is afterward filled with healing tissue whose properties are different from the corneal tissue.

Some surgical techniques use variations in incision depth to obtain different refractive changes. The radial keratotomy for myopia, the Lindstrom arcuate technique for astigmatism, and the Arciniegas parallel technique for myopia and astigmatism are simulated [14]. These techniques perform incisions to maximum depth (90–95 % of the corneal thickness).

3.2 Generation of a Curvature Map

The structural analysis allows to observe geometrical changes and stress concentration zones. However, the ophthalmologist evaluates the surgical results from refractive changes in the corneal structure. Usually, he verifies the refractive changes by measuring the corneal curvatures with the keratometer, an optical instrument that measures four points at the corneal central zone and determines curvature from the sphere–cylindrical assumption of the corneal shape.

By incorporating a map of corneal curvatures, the refractive surgery can be analyzed broader (Fig. 3.2). The corneal topography allows the detection of irregular astigmatism appearing after the surgery. In addition, the paracentral and peripheral surgical effect is visible.

The axial curvature radius is calculated by fitting a circumference with three successive points in a meridian. By this way, we are able to compare the corneal topography after a surgical simulation with that measured after a real surgery, allowing to validate the model 3 y 4. This method is more powerful than those employed in other works [17–20] which calculated refractive changes in the cornea, by fitting an ellipsoid or paraboloid in the central zone (limiting the analysis to patients with regular astigmatism) [21].

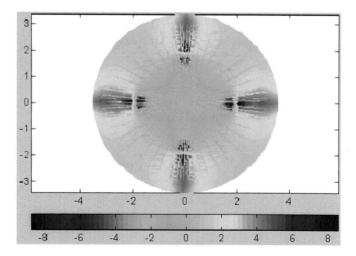

Fig. 3.2 After finite element analysis, a topographical map is calculated from the deformed shape. In the color plot, it is shown the difference in refraction from the presurgery map. The central zone shows a negative change of -2 D (flattening). In the incisions, the refractive change is higher

4 Parametric Study of Radial Keratotomy

In order to validate the proposed technique, we first studied the sensitivity of a simulation of 4-incision radial keratotomy to variations in the intraocular pressure; surgical parameters, i.e., the incision length, the optical zone diameter, and the incision depth; and material parameters, i.e., Young's modulus and Poisson's ratio. We intended to validate with clinical and experimental results. In Fig. 3.9 it is shown the finite element mesh of the simulated 4-incisions radial keratotomy and the modulus of displacement is represented by a colored scale.

4.1 Relation with the Incision Length

The changes in curvature with variations in incision length were analyzed, by regarding the curvature radius in the astigmatism axes (0°, 90°) at 0.7 mm from the apex (Fig. 3.3). The optical zone was 2 mm, and four radial incisions were performed in the axes 0°, 90°, 180°, and 270°.

In general, a change in the length of the incision produces a change in the refraction by increasing the radius of curvature (flattening) in the central zone. The change decreases with longer incisions.

4.2 Relation with the Optical Zone

For a 7 mm incision length, the optical zone diameter was varied from 3 to 4 mm. We did not find a substantial change for incision of equal length having different clear zones between 3 and 4 mm in diameter.

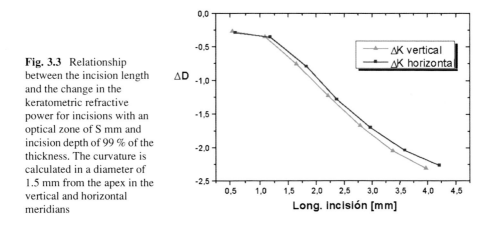

Fig. 3.3 Relationship between the incision length and the change in the keratometric refractive power for incisions with an optical zone of S mm and incision depth of 99 % of the thickness. The curvature is calculated in a diameter of 1.5 mm from the apex in the vertical and horizontal meridians

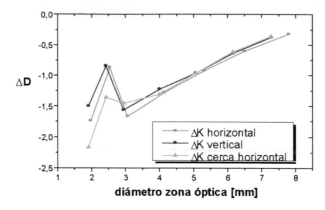

Fig. 3.4 Relationship between the diameter of the optical zone and the change in the keratometric refractive power for incisions with an incision length of 2.3 mm and incision depth of 99 % of the thickness. The curvature is calculated in a diameter of 1.5 mm from the apex in the vertical and horizontal meridians. For an optical zone lower than 2.5 mm, the incision produces distortion in the calculation of the keratometric curvature

We found a decrease in the refractive change when increasing the optical zone as expected (Fig. 3.4). Results were compared with the work of Pinsky et al. [20]. We found a general agreement in medium and large optical zones, but results differed for the smallest optical zone case since we are measuring the keratometric curvature which employs five points (2 in horizontal meridian, 2 in vertical meridian, 1 at apex) to calculate curvature instead of a spherical within a 3.00 mm zone used by Pinsky et al. [20].

4.3 Relation with Incision Depth

The increase in the incision depth produces greater flattening, almost linearly by the four-incision pattern (Fig. 3.5). Increasing the number of incisions would produce nonlinear variations. The elastic modulus and Poisson's ratio were 3 MPa and 0.45, respectively.

4.4 Effect of the Young's Modulus

We varied Young's modulus from 0.6 to 15 MPa, in the eyes with 4 radial incisions. The Poisson's ratio was 0.45. We present in Fig. 3.6 the radius of curvature measured in the apex, 3 and 5 mm from the apex vs. the elastic moduli in MPa.

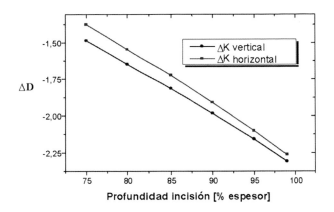

Fig. 3.5 Relationship between the incision depth and the change in the keratometric refractive power for incisions with an optical zone of S mm and incision length of U mm. The curvature is calculated in a diameter of 1.5 mm, from the apex in the vertical and horizontal meridians

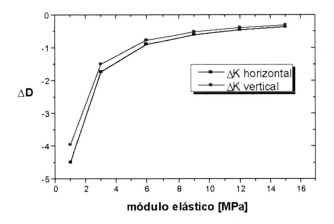

Fig. 3.6 Relationship between the elastic modulus and the change in the keratometric refractive power for incisions with an optical zone of S mm, incision length of U mm, and incision depth of 99 % of the thickness. The curvature is calculated in a diameter of 1.5 mm from the apex in the vertical and horizontal meridians. For stiffer corneas (older), the effect of the surgery is low

We found the lower the elastic modulus, the greater the correction. For values of elastic modulus greater than 11 MPa, the correction is smaller. This could be correlated with the stiffening age dependence reported [14].

4.5 Relation with the Poisson's Ratio

The variation with the Poisson's ratio was studied (Fig. 3.7). We found a negligible effect of the Poisson's ratio from 0.2 to 0.4. The elastic modulus was 3 MPa.

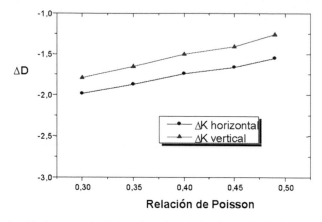

Fig. 3.7 Relationship between the Poisson's ratio and the change in the keratometric refractive power for incisions with an optical zone of 2 mm, incision length of 2.3 mm, and incision depth of 99 % of the thickness. The curvature is calculated in a diameter of 1.5 mm, from the apex in the vertical and horizontal meridians

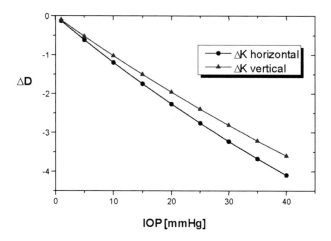

Fig. 3.8 Relationship between the intraocular pressure and the change in the keratometric refractive power for incisions with an optical zone of 2 mm, incision length of 2.3 mm, and incision depth of 99 % of the thickness. The curvature is calculated in a diameter of 1.5 mm from the apex in the vertical and horizontal meridians

4.6   Relation with Intraocular Pressure

It was found that the effect of surgery increases with the intraocular pressure (Fig. 3.8). High eye pressures (>25 mmHg, like in glaucoma) present changes of 1–2D greater than in the physiological range (15–20 mmHg). The elastic modulus and Poisson's ratio were 3 MPa and 0.45, respectively.

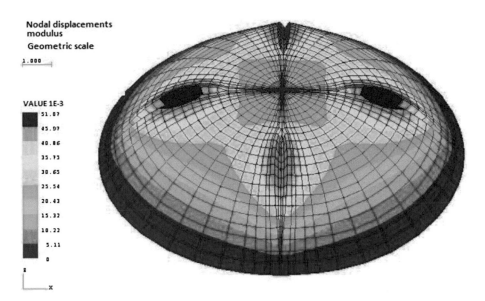

Nodal displacements modulus

Geometric scale

1.000

VALUE 1E-3

- 51.07
- 45.97
- 40.86
- 35.73
- 30.63
- 25.54
- 20.43
- 15.32
- 10.22
- 5.11
- 0

Fig. 3.9 A colored graphic representation of the modulus of displacement (factor scale × 15). The horizontal incision gap is more pronounced than the vertical ones because of the different corneal diameters

5 Discussion

In this work, a structural model of the human cornea based on the finite element method was described. SAMCEF was used to perform the model preparation and the linear static analysis.

The geometrical model of the cornea considered in this work describes any type of ametropias, as well as any kind of pathologies which alter the corneal geometry. There were not geometrical assumptions, like symmetry axes, or revolution surfaces. Structural parameters resulting from a material homogenization performed by Hanna et al. were used. It was considered a linear behavior of the material binding analysis to low intraocular pressure (13–20 mmHg, which is the range of normal pressure for the surgical technique). By considering only a static analysis, the variations in the corneal parameters over time are not taken into account. Further studies about the wound healing process are necessary.

The size of the mesh, as well as the local effect sensitivity, was determined with a criterion to minimize the computational cost. Due to the expensive cost of this technique, the reduction in the analysis time allowed the study of the variations of several parameters.

The refractive results of the variation of the characteristic parameters of the model determined that it behaves acceptably well, imitating the real behavior of the cornea at the same conditions. The result of comparing the simulation with a real surgery only confirmed the previous conclusion. The error was greater than the desirable (± 0.25 D).

Although there are many considerations, the main sources of the difference could be assigned to the boundary conditions imposed, data measuring errors, and an insufficient refinement of the mesh. The last factor could explain the stiffness showed by the numerical model.

At the point of view of the numerical model, we estimate convenience to incorporate error estimation strategies and an automatic mesh refinement to represent adequately the strong gradients introduced in the incisions. Similarly, we estimate the necessity to perform a better validation of the material behavior model of the corneal tissue (i.e., in the prior months to surgery, a refractive change that could be associated to a relaxation phenomenon was observed).

The results of this study are part of an interdisciplinary work between physicians and engineers. By integrating different contributions of the disciplines, like the engineering and the medicine, it is possible to reach fruitful results in the biomedical research area.

6   An Exponential Hyperelastic Material Model for the Corneal Tissue

The biomechanical response of the cornea *in surgical procedures* has been described mostly for radial keratotomy by measuring local deformations [22–24]. Others have used finite element models with different assumptions regarding corneal geometry and material properties. Some have assumed that the cornea is a homogeneous linear elastic solid [21, 25, 26], nonlinear elastic [17, 24, 27, 28] solid, and a nonhomogeneous membrane [20].

Attempts to verify the models have been done with inflation tests [28] in hydrated corneas and with local deformations [24] in normo-hydrated corneas. The relationship between corneal strain and intraocular pressure was found to be nonlinear, showing a typical stress-stiffening behavior. A material model by Woo et al. [12] has been used to account that nonlinearity [24, 27, 28].

The anisotropy of the cornea is evidenced by its microstructure as a reinforced composite with collagen fibers immersed in a jellylike matrix of mucopolysaccharides. There have been attempts to account the anisotropy of the cornea, with transverse isotropy but since the cornea is also nearly incompressible [29] violates the restrictions on the elastic constants [Sutcu 1992]. Pinsky et al. modeled the anisotropy produced by the relaxing incisions in a thick membrane model. But local bending effects near the incision were found to be an important factor [23].

The hydration has a profound effect on the extensibility of the stroma [23], and viscoelastic properties have been measured in vivo after radial keratotomy [30].

A complete model of the cornea should take into account the poroelasticity, viscoelasticity, and anisotropicity of the cornea.

Hyperelastic models are appropriate for material and geometrical nonlinearities. Geometric nonlinearities appear in inflation tests as well as in refractive procedures like those involving the insertion of intrastromal rings. They are also suitable for further extension to anisotropy and inelasticity. There were attempts to use rubber-based hyperelastic models, like Mooney–Rivlin [28, 31] and Ogden [28], but they did not reproduce the high nonlinearity of the cornea.

A hyperelastic model is presented that accounts for the nonlinearity of the cornea, both material and geometrical, and is suitable for viscoelasticity [32] and poroelasticity. Inflations tests [28, 33] are proposed in hydrated and normo-hydrated corneas to obtain the material parameters of the model.

7 Exponential Models for Biological Tissues

Several authors proposed to use exponential material models to represent the nonlinear elastic behavior of biological tissues. For instance, Fung proposed the following strain energy:

$$W = \frac{\mu_0}{2\gamma}\left[e^{\gamma(I_1 - 3)} - 1\right] \tag{3.2}$$

where μ_0 (shear modulus) and seven are positive material constants [34, 35]. Also, Woo et al. [12] used an exponential model, in small strains, to analyze the corneal stroma, sclera, and optic nerve:

$$\sigma_{\text{eff}} = \alpha\left(e^{\beta\varepsilon_{\text{eff}}} - 1\right) \tag{3.3}$$

where σ_{eff} and ε_{eff} *are* effective stress and strain, respectively, and α and β *are* material constants. Bryant et al. used a similar model and characterized its parameters in an inflation test after failing with the Mooney-Rivlin and Ogden models. This model accounts for the material nonlinearity but is not suitable for further developments of viscoelasticity, as it was proposed in [32].

7.1 Hyperelastic Nearly Incompressible Exponential Model for the Cornea

A hyperelastic exponential model is proposed, with an integral of the exponential term, in order to have a simpler form in the stress and elasticity matrix, after differentiation. A second logarithmic term is added with the second invariant of the deformation tensor C (similar to the Hart–Smith model) and a third logarithmic term with the third invariant of the deformation tensor C to account the near incompressibility [36, 37].

The strain energy function W results in

$$W(I_1, I_2, I_3) = c_1 \int e^{c_3(I_1-3)} dI_1 + c_2 \ln\frac{I_2}{3} + 2c_4(I_3 - 1) + c_5(\ln I_3)^2 \quad (3.4)$$

with material constants c_1, c_2, c_3, c_4, and c_5.

The second tensor of Piola–Kirchhoff is now

$$\mathbf{S} = 2\partial_C W(\mathbf{C}) = 2\left(c_1 e^{c_3(I_1-3)} + \frac{c_2 I_1}{I_2}\right)\mathbf{1} - 2\frac{c_2}{I_2}\mathbf{C} + 4(c_4 I_3 + c_5 \ln(I_3))\mathbf{C}^{-1} \quad (3.5)$$

The nonzero principal value of the first Piola-Kirchhoff stress tensor P_{11} in a simple tension test of an incompressible exponential hyperelastic material may be written as follows:

$$P_{11} = 2\left(1 - \frac{1}{\lambda^3}\right)\left(c_1 \lambda e^{c_3\left(\lambda^2 + 2\lambda^{-1} - 3\right)} + \frac{c_2}{2\lambda + \lambda^{-2}}\right) \quad (3.6)$$

Parameters c_1, c_2, and c_3 are then adjusted to match the curve $P_{11}(\lambda)$ observed in the test.

This material has been implemented using the finite element methods [38].

7.1.1 Fitting Inflation Tests Using an Inverse Method

From inflation tests with corneas from human enucleated eyes [28], the material parameters of the exponential model were fitted. An inverse method was used to reproduce intraocular pressure Pjq vs. apical displacement d_{apical} experimental curves. The test was modeled as an axisymmetric structure using finite elements, with the symmetry axis oriented along the anterior–posterior axis of the eye and dimensions taken from the paper of Bryant et al. (Fig. 3.10). The mesh consisted of

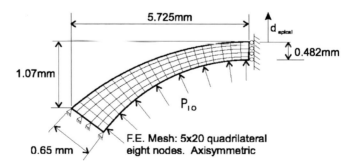

Fig. 3.10 Axisymmetric finite element mesh used to model the inflation test of Bryant et al. The corneal radius was 5.725 mm; the thickness at the apex was 0.482 mm and at the limbus 0.65 mm. The intraocular pressure (IOP) was 15 mmHg and the apical height of the cornea was 1.07 mm

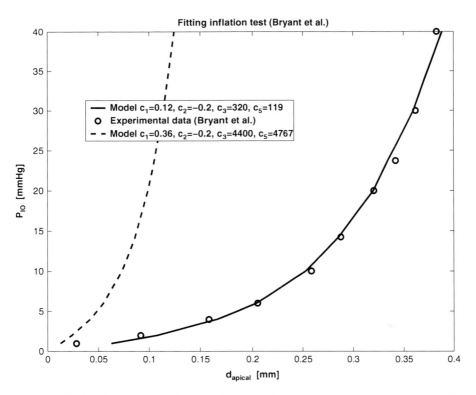

Fig. 3.11 Fitting the experimental curve of the inflation test with an exponential hyperelastic model by means of an inverse method

five layers of finite elements with quadratic interpolation and was refined to give enough accurate results for the problem.

A nonlinear optimization algorithm, originally implemented by R. Hooke and T. A. Jeeves [39], was used to fit parameters. The process started taking as initial values the parameters obtained when fitting the derived pure tension curve.

There was good agreement with the experimental curve $P_{IO} - d_{\mathrm{apical}}$ (Fig. 3.11).

7.1.2 Fitting Normo-Hydrated Inflation Tests

The extensibility of ten human corneas was evaluated in vitro by Hjortdal [33]. The central epithelial side strain was measured, induced by intraocular pressure loads ranging from 2 to 100 mmHg. Corneal normo-hydration was attempted by immersing and perfusing the eyes with 8 % Dextran 500 in isotonic saline. The relation between corneal strain and intraocular pressure was found to be strongly nonlinear, showing a typical stress-stiffening behavior. Compared with previous experiments

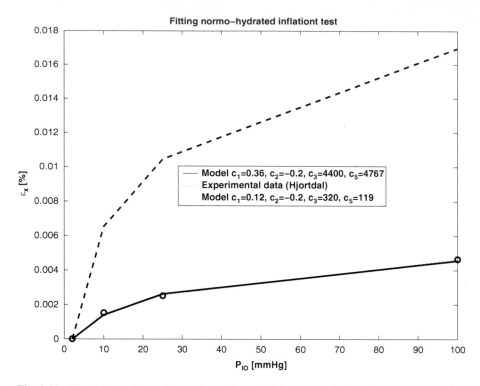

Fig. 3.12 Hjortdal experimental curve for strain vs. IOP in a normo-hydrated cornea compared to the computed curve with optimal material parameters

performed with swollen corneas, the stiffness of the normo-hydrated human cornea was found to be higher.

The material parameters, that is, the experimentally measured IOP-epithelial side strain curve, were obtained using an axisymmetric model including the limbus and sclera as shown in Fig. 3.12 where a comparison of the measured and simulated curves is shown.

7.2   Simulation of Radial Keratotomy

In addition to the regional strain patterns due to IOP, Hjortdal et al. studied the regional deformation pattern of the cornea after radial keratotomy [15]. The hydration was controlled in this experiment with a solution of 8 % Dextran T500 in 0.9 % NaCl for preserving the corneal thickness. In this experiment, four radial incisions were made with a double-edged diamond knife. The incisor depth was set to 100 %

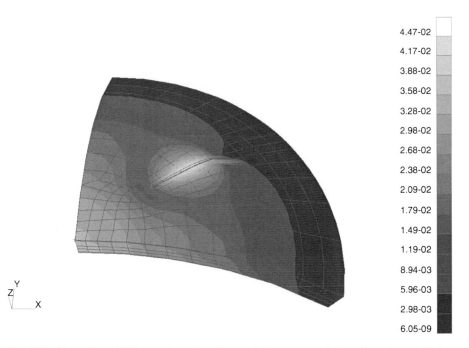

4.47-02
4.17-02
3.88-02
3.58-02
3.28-02
2.98-02
2.68-02
2.38-02
2.09-02
1.79-02
1.49-02
1.19-02
8.94-03
5.96-03
2.98-03
6.05-09

Y
Z
X

Fig. 3.13 Simulation of RK experiment based on model parameters obtained from intact inflation tests

of the central corneal thickness. The central optical zone was 3.5 mm. The incision was made from the center toward the periphery with subsequent re-deepening. After the completion of the experiments, it was checked that the incisions penetrated to more than 90 % of the corneal thickness by histology.

The radial keratotomy induced 2.30 D of central flattening at an intraocular pressure of 2 mmHg. In the physiological pressure range, the central cornea flattened 0.05 D for each mmHg in intraocular pressure. The degree of central flattening correlated linearly with the amount of wound gape.

We used 3D isoparametric solid elements with four layers of elements across the thickness of the cornea. The mesh was refined at the incision zones. It was introduced as boundary conditions, the limbus and sclera. A portion of the sclera and a transition zone with the limbus were modeled. The degrees of freedom were fixed in the y direction, parallel to the visual axis [18].

A typical result for the 3D RK model is shown in Fig. 3.13, where the contours indicate change in the z contour.

In Fig. 3.14, we plot the flattening at the apex.

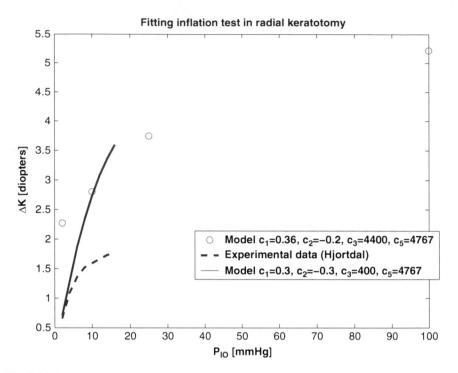

Fig. 3.14 Hjortdal experimental curve for flattening in diopters vs. IOP in a normo-hydrated cornea compared to the computed curve with material parameters

Concluding Remarks

We have presented a constitutive model for biological tissues with high nonlinearity, appropriate to describe the mechanical behavior of the human cornea. The model was developed in the context of a finite elasticity formulation. This *exponential hyperelastic material model* was derived from the Hart–Smith model and tested in both the axisymmetric and tridimensional cases. Explicit expressions for the symmetric Piola–Kirchhoff stress tensor and for the tangent modulus were given.

We have made a series of tests to validate the use of this model and performed comparisons with other material models mentioned in the literature. The exponential hyperelastic material model was able to represent accurately either experiments performed on corneal strips (simple tension tests) or on intact eyes (inflation tests) matching satisfactorily the P_{IO} vs d_{apical} experimental curve. The obtained parameters represented the behavior of the cornea for a wide range of variation of the intraocular pressure. On the other hand, material models such as Mooney–Rivlin and Hart–Smith failed when representing one or another test, confirming observations made by other

(continued)

(continued)

authors [28]. This model also behaves well in compression. It has been found
[29] that the sclera presents an exponential behavior in compression. No data
is available for the cornea. We assumed that the tissue behaves similarly in
low tension and low compression, where the elasticity of the ground substance is more important than the wavy collagen fibers. For higher compressive stresses, where the wavy collagen fibers are collapsed, we expect a
different behavior than in high tension where the fibers are stretched. In radial
keratotomy and lamellar procedures, the compressive forces are low.

The exponential hyperelastic model gave results higher with those
expected from the surgery, both for refractive changes and incision opening.
The test indicates that properly accounting for the material and geometrical
nonlinearities is of utmost importance for accurately modeling this surgery.
Given the in vitro nature of the inflation tests, where the corneas could have
been more hydrated than in the physiological state, we assumed than the
parameters obtained from these tests are from the softer corneas than normal.
We could have modified the material parameters until we get the desirable
results for RK, but we are not interested in having good results with a
particular case but to real calibrate the material. This goal will enable us to
use this model with other procedures like PRK and LASIK.

The proposed constitutive model of the cornea allows to account for large
strains and material nonlinearity, characteristic of biological tissue. Extension
of this model to orthotropic materials would allow to analyze many hydrated
soft tissues with high nonlinearity such as the skin, tendons, and ligaments.

The model developed may be used for other ophthalmological applications, such as the simulation of photokeratectomy and keratomileusis.
Although in the examples we only presented incisional refractive surgery
applications, other surgical techniques like PRK and LASIK may be also
analyzed and will be addressed in the next chapter.

8   Finite Linear Viscoelastic Model

In order to simulate the viscoelastic effect in the cornea after a refractive procedure,
a 3D finite element was developed in large strains.

The viscoelastic effects of the cornea have been measured in inflations tests [40],
in corneal strips [Seiler 1992], and in cylindrical corneal samples [41]. In vivo
properties were measured by Buzard et al. after refractive procedures [30].

The theory of quasilinear viscoelasticity proposed by Fung has been widely used
to describe the viscoelastic behavior of soft tissues but lacks of a consistent
molecular theory.

Lubliner assumed a multiplicative decomposition of the deformation gradient
into elastic and inelastic parts and interpreted the theory of relaxation effects

from Green and Tobolsky in a self-consistent molecular theory of rubbers. This multiplicative decomposition was applied in nonlinear viscoelasticity by Sidoroff. In this theory, a large deformation was taken into account, but small deviations from the thermodynamic equilibrium were assumed. In this case, the theory is called finite linear viscoelasticity.

Many implementations of finite viscoelasticity use for the equilibrium and nonequilibrium parts of the material model the class of Ogden models that agree with experimental results in rubbers. Bryant et al. [28] showed that this class of models is not appropriate to reproduce membranal inflation test of the human corneas nor rubber-based hyperelastic models. Le Tallec used simple hyperelastic models for both parts to model the cornea and radial keratotomy. Bryant et al. suggested the importance of the material nonlinearity of the cornea for a model of refractive surgery. Guarnieri et al. [32] presented an exponential hyperelastic model that accounts for the high nonlinearity of the human cornea with large strains.

In the next section, a finite linear viscoelastic model is described using for the equilibrium part the exponential hyperelastic model for the human cornea and a simple hyperelastic model for the nonequilibrium part.

9 Constitutive Equations

In Fig. 3.15, we shown schematically the standard linear viscoelastic solid or Kelvin model [42] as combined by linear springs with elastic constants $/i$ and $/iq$ and a dashpot with a viscosity constant 77.

In analogy to the linear viscoelasticity in small strain, we can assume an additive free energy potential with the form

$$W(\mathbf{C}, \mathbf{C}_v) = W_0(\mathbf{C}) + W_e(\mathbf{C}_e) \tag{3.7}$$

where W_0 measures the energy stored in the elastic branch (equilibrium) and W_e measures the energy stored in the viscous branch, which progressively disappears

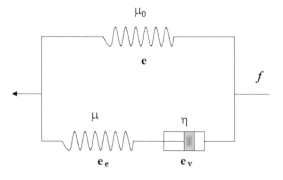

Fig. 3.15 The standard linear viscoelastic solid or Kelvin model

during the relaxation. In large strains, the right Cauchy–Green tensors $\mathbf{C}$, $\mathbf{C}_e$, and $\mathbf{C}_v$ measure the total deformation, the elastic part, and the viscous part in the viscoelastic branch, respectively. The tensor $\mathbf{C}_v$ *is an* internal viscoelastic variable.

A dissipation function is postulated in the dashpot that satisfies the Clausius–Duhem (second thermodynamic law) inequality:

$$\phi(\dot{\mathbf{C}}_v) : \dot{\mathbf{C}}_v \geq 0 \tag{3.8}$$

9.1 Multiplicative Decomposition of the Deformation Gradient

The additive decomposition of the deformation is not appropriate in large strains. In this case, the multiplicative decomposition is used. The total gradient deformation gradient F is split into an elastic part $\mathbf{F}_e$ and an inelastic (or viscous) part $\mathbf{F}_v$, resulting to

$$\begin{aligned}
\mathbf{F} &= \mathbf{F}_e\mathbf{F}_v \\
\mathbf{C} &= \mathbf{F}_v^T\mathbf{C}_e\mathbf{F}_v \\
J &= J_eJ_v
\end{aligned} \tag{3.9}$$

where $J = \det(\mathrm{F}) > 0$.

9.2 Finite Linear Viscoelasticity

Applying the first principle of thermodynamics in an isothermal process, we have

$$dissipated\ heat = work - free\ energy(9) \tag{3.10}$$

Then, in a reference configuration, we have

$$\phi(\dot{\mathbf{C}}_v) : d\mathbf{C}_v = \frac{1}{2}\mathbf{S} : d\mathbf{C} - dW \tag{3.11}$$

where $\mathbf{S}$ is the symmetric Piola–Kirchhoff tensor. Given that the state variables $\mathbf{C}$ and $\mathbf{C}_v$ are supposed to be independent, then

$$\begin{aligned}
\mathbf{S} &= 2\frac{\partial W(\mathbf{C}, \mathbf{C}_v)}{\partial \mathbf{C}} \\
\phi(\dot{\mathbf{C}}_v) &= -\frac{\partial W(\mathbf{C}, \mathbf{C}_v)}{\partial \mathbf{C}_v}
\end{aligned} \tag{3.12}$$

The first equation is the hyperelastic constitutive law with $\mathbf{C}_v$ as a constitutive parameter. The second equation is a first-order differential equation where the variable $\mathbf{C}_v$ introduces the dependence with time in the model.

This model is motivated by experimental data, where time-dependent change in the free energy is only due to isochoric deformations.

To describe the viscoelastic response, we choose the exponential hyperelastic model as the energy function Wq for the equilibrium response and a simple hyperelastic model with an energy function W_e for the nonequilibrium branch:

$$W(\mathbf{C}, \mathbf{C}_v) = W_0(\mathbf{E}) + W_e(\mathbf{C}_e)$$
$$W_0(\mathbf{E}) = c_1 \int e^{c_3(I_1-3)} dI_1 + c_2 \ln\frac{I_2}{3} + 2c_4(I_3 - 1) + c_5(\ln I_3)^2 \qquad (3.13)$$
$$W_e(\mathbf{C}_e) = W_1(tr\mathbf{C}_e) + W_2(det\mathbf{C}_e)$$

We choose

$$\phi(\dot{\mathbf{C}}_v) = -\eta \frac{\dot{}}{\mathbf{C}_v^{-1}}$$

where η is a positive definite, symmetric viscosity tensor. This model was implemented using the finite element method [38].

9.3 Calibration with In Vivo Corneal Experiment

In order to reproduce the experimental curves of the recovering creep in the work of Buzard [30], a finite element model of the cornea was considered. An initial intraocular pressure of 30 mmHg, equivalent to the pressure produced by the Honan balloon used in the experiment, was set. Once obtained, the equilibrium response, the IOP, was recovered to its physiological value of 15 mmHg.

In the linearized model, the secant modulus, that is, the curve IOP vs. the apical displacement in the Bryant's experiment, was calculated iteratively for 30 and 15 mmHg with a Poisson's ratio of $u = 0.48$ (Table 3.1). The value of the elastic modulus for the instantaneous response was considered using the estimated value of Edmund [43] of 9 MPa.

An 8-node, solid, finite element mesh was used consisting of four layers with 20×20 elements in each layer.

Table 3.1 Table with the values of IOP and apical displacement in the simulation of the corneal inflation

Model	IOP [mmHg]	d. apical [mm]	Young's modulus [MPa]
Exp. Bryant et al.	15	0.29	0.789 (tangent)
Exp. Bryant et al.	30	0.36	–
LDT10/linear interp.	15	0.2908	0.88
LDT10/linear interp.	30	0.3622	1.31

Tangent and secant moduli are also shown per IOP

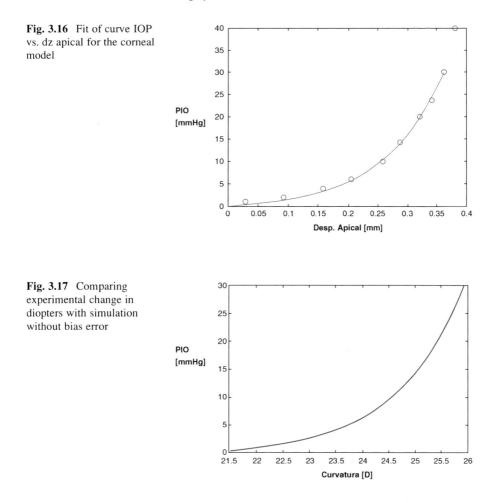

Fig. 3.16 Fit of curve IOP vs. dz apical for the corneal model

Fig. 3.17 Comparing experimental change in diopters with simulation without bias error

Table 3.2 Material parameters of the exponential hyperelastic model

C1	C2	C3	C5	Norm (e)
0.05	0	1000	388	0.0463

The experimental curve IOP vs. d_{z_apical} *is* fitted as it is shown in Figs. 3.16 and 3.17. The material parameters of the exponential hyperelastic model are presented in Table 3.2.

Comparing the experimental curve from Buzard et al., the error of the nonlinear viscoelastic model with the exponential hyperelastic model was lower than 0.4 D (Fig. 3.18). This error was calculated after releasing the pressure of the Honan balloon (30 mmHg) and subtracting the bias error presented in the Buzard experiment (see details in [38]).

Fig. 3.18 Comparing experimental change in diopters with simulation without bias error

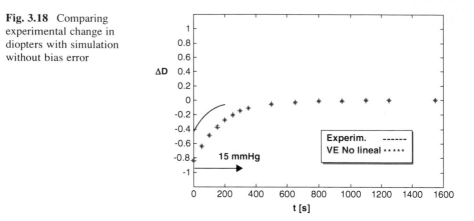

Conclusions

In this work, a formulation of a 3D nonlinear viscoelastic finite element was described which combines an exponential hyperelastic model for the human cornea.

The simulation of the experimental IOP increase with a Honan balloon performed by Buzard et al. coincides approximately with the experiment (without bias error or baseline error). This error was 0.4 D. Since there are several uncertainties like the elastic properties of the in vivo corneas used in the experiment, the geometry, and the estimated value used for the instantaneous modulus (9 ± 0.42 MPa), we cannot assure the final error.

References

1. G.O. Waring III, Making sense of 'keratospeak'. A classification of refractive corneal surgery. Arch. Ophthalmol. **103**(10), 1472–77 (1985)
2. W. Ellis, *Radial Keratotomy and Astigmatism Surgery* (Medical Aesthetics Inc., Newport Beach, 1986)
3. S. Mandelbaum, M. Lynn, Radial keratotomy. From the Prospective Evaluation of Radial Keratotomy (PERK), Clinical Center at the Bascom Palmer Eye Institute, University of Florida and the Biostatistical Coordinating Center at Emory University, Atlanta, Georgia, 1985
4. R.A. Villaseñor, G.R. Stimac, Clinical results and complications of trapezoidal keratotomy. J. Refract. Surg. **4**, 125–131 (1988)
5. Board of Directors of the International Society of Refractive Keratoplasty, Statement on radial keratotomy in 1988. J. Refract. Surg. **4**, 80–90 (1988)
6. M.J. Lynn, G.O. Waring, R.D. Sperduto, the PERK Study Group, Factors affecting outcome and predictability of radial keratotomy in the perk study. Arch Ophthalmol. **105**, 42–51 (1987)
7. O.C. Zienkiewicz, R.L. Taylor, *The Finite Element Method*, 1st edn. (McGraw-Hill, Barcelona, 1994)
8. J. Engelstein, *Cirugía de las Cataratas. Ed,* 2nd edn. (Panamericana, Bs. As., 1985)
9. D. Christensen, *Ultrasonic Bioinstrumentation* (Wiley, New York, 1988)

10. D. Schanzlin, J. Robin, *Corneal Topography. Measuring and Modifying the Cornea* (Springer, New York, 1992)
11. J. Gloster, E.S. Perkins, M.-L. Pommier, Extensibility of strips of sclera and cornea. British. J. Ophthal. **41**, 103–110 (1957)
12. S.L.-Y. Woo, A.S. Kobayashi, W.A. Schlegel, C. Lawrence, Nonlinear material properties of intact cornea and sclera. Exp. Eye Res. **14**, 29–39 (1972)
13. P.R. Greene, T.A. McMahon, Scleral creep vs. temperature and pressure in vitro. Exp. Eye Res. **29**, 527–537 (1979)
14. A. Arciniegas, L.E. Amaya, *Asociación de la queratotomía radial y la circular para la corrección de* ametropias. *Enfoque biomecánico,* chapter XXII. Soc. Am. de Oftalmología, Bogotá, 1981
15. I.S. Nash, P.R. Greene, C.S. Foster, Comparison of mechanical properties of keratoconus and normal corneas. Exp. Eye Res. **35**, 413–423 (1982)
16. B. Jue, D. Maurice, The mechanical properties of the rabbit and human cornea. J. Biomech. **19** (10), 847–854 (1986)
17. K.D. Hanna, F.E. Jouve, G.O. Waring III, Computer simulation of arcuate keratotomy for astigmatism. Refract. Corneal Surg. **8**(2), 152–163 (1992)
18. P.H. Carnell, R.P. Vito, A model for estimating corneal stiffness using an indenter. J. Biomech. Eng. **114**(4), 549–552 (1992)
19. M.R. Sawusch, P.J. McDonnell, Computer modeling of wound gape following radial keratotomy. Refract. Corneal Surg. **8**(2), 143–145 (1992)
20. P.M. Pinsky, D.V. Datye, Numerical modeling of radial, astigmatic and hexagonal keratotomy. Refract. Corneal Surg. **8**(2), 164–172 (1992)
21. F.A. Guarnieri, Modelo biomecánico del ojo para diseño asistido por computadora de la cirugía refractiva. Proyecto de grado de bioingeniería, Facultad de Ingeniería, UNER, Oro Verde, Entre Ríos, Argentina, 1993
22. K.A. Buzard, J.F. Ronk, M.H. Friedlander, D.J. Tepper, D.A. Hoeltzel, K. Choe, Quantitative measurement of wound spreading in radial keratotomy. Refract. Corneal Surg. **8**(3), 217–223 (1992)
23. J.O. Hjortdal, N. Ehlers, Acute tissue deformation of the human cornea after radial keratotomy. J. Refract. Surg. **12**(3), 391–400 (1996)
24. W.M. Petroll, P. Roy, C.J. Chuong, B. Hall, H.D. Cavanagh, J.V. Jester, Measurement of surgically induced corneal deformations using three-dimensional confocal microscopy. Cornea **15**(2), 154–164 (1996)
25. R.P. Vito, P.H. Carnell, Finite element method based mechanical models of the cornea for pressure and indenter loading. Refract. Corneal Surg. **8**(2), 146–151 (1992)
26. S.C. Velinsky, M.R. Bryant, On the computer-aided and optimal design of keratorefractive surgery. Refract. Corneal Surg. **8**(2), 173–182 (1992)
27. W.O. Wray, E.D. Best, L.Y. Cheng, A mechanical model for radial keratotomy: toward a predictive capability. J. Biomech. Eng. **116**(1), 56–61 (1994)
28. M.R. Bryant, P.J. McDonnell, Constitutive laws for biomechanical modeling of refractive surgery. J. Biomech. Eng. **118**, 473–481 (1996)
29. J.L. Battaglioli, R.D. Kamm, Measurements of the compressive properties of scleral tissue. Invest. Ophthalmol. Vis. Sci. **114**(2), 202–215 (1992)
30. K.A. Buzard, B.R. Fundingsland, Assessment of corneal wound healing by interactive topography. J. Refract. Surg. **14**, 53–60 (1998)
31. K.D. Hanna, F.E. Jouve, G.O. Waring III, Preliminary computer simulation of the effects of radial keratotomy. Arch. Ophthalmol. **107**, 911–918 (1989)
32. F.A. Guarnieri, A. Cardona, 3d viscoelastic nonlinear incompressible finite element in large strain of the cornea. application in refractive surgery, in *Articles in CD-ROM Fourth World Congress of Computational Mechanics,* 1998
33. J.O. Hjortdal, N. Ehlers, Extensibility of the normo-hydrated human cornea. Acta Ophthalmol. Scand. **73**(1), 12–17 (1995)

34. M.F. Beatty, Topics in finite elasticity: hyperelasticity of rubber, elastomers, and biological tissues – with examples. Appl. Mech Rev. **40**, 1699–1734 (1987)
35. Y.C. Fung, *Biomechanics. Mechanical Properties of Living Tissues*, 2nd edn. (Springer, New York, 1993)
36. A.D. Drozdov, *Finite Elasticity and Viscoelasticity. A Course in the Nonlinear Mechanics of Solids* (World Scientific, Singapore, 1996)
37. Samtech. The *SAMCEF User's Manuals – V7.1*. Samtech, Liége,á Belgium, silver edition, 4.
38. F.A. Guarnieri, Modelo Biomecánico del Ojo para Diseño Asistido por Computadora de la Cirugía Refractiva. PhD dissertation, FICH-INTEC, Universidad Nacional del Litoral, Santa Fe, Argentina, 1999
39. M.G. Johnson. Nonlinear Optimization using the algorithm of Hooke and Jeeves, 1994. Documentación en código fuente en C.
40. A.S. Kobayashi, L.G. Staberg, W.A. Schlegel, Viscoelastic properties of human cornea. Exp. Mech. **13**(12), 497–503 (1973)
41. M.K. Smolek, Holographic interferometry of intact and radially incised human eye-bank corneas. J. Cataract Refract. Surg. **20**, 277–286 (1994)
42. R.M. Christensen, *Theory de viscoelasticity: An Introduction* (Academic, New York, 1971)
43. C. Edmund, Corneal topography and elasticity in normal and keratoconic eyes. Acta Ophthalmol. **193**, 1–36 (1989)

Chapter 4
Biomechanics of Subtractive Surgery: From ALK to LASIK

Fabio A. Guarnieri

1 Introduction

Myopic and hyperopic excimer laser in situ keratomileusis (LASIK) have become widely accepted procedures. Although LASIK does not rely on the mechanical response of the cornea to obtain the optical correction, the creation of a flap and ablation of the exposed stromal bed must disturb the state of stress in the tissue below the ablation zone. Little attention appears to have been paid to the mechanical response of the cornea to LASIK [1–3]. For low to moderate correction, the stress change induced by the surgical procedure is probably relatively small, although, it has not been quantified to date. As interest moves to deeper ablation depths, it is increasingly important to understand the mechanical response of the tissue to its new geometric configuration. Clearly, as ablation depths vary from shallow to very deep, the cornea can be expected to exhibit a corresponding range of deformational responses. The deformational response of the cornea to LASIK can be identified with an instantaneous component associated with the intrinsic elasticity of the tissue and a delayed postoperative component that may be associated with possible regression and that derives from complex and poorly understood mechanisms.

A finite element model for analyzing the instantaneous response of the cornea to LASIK is outlined below. In addition to providing insight into the parameters that control the structural response of the cornea to LASIK, the model could also shed some light on the question of what constitutes a safe minimum posterior stromal bed thickness.

F.A. Guarnieri, Ph.D. (✉)
Department of Bioengineering, Centro de Investigación de Métodos
Computacionales (CIMEC), Predio CONICET-Santa Fe, Colectora Ruta Nac 168,
Km 472, Paraje El Pozo, 3000 Santa Fe, Argentina
e-mail: aguarni@santafe-conicet.gov.ar

© Springer Science+Business Media New York 2015   57
F.A. Guarnieri (ed.), *Corneal Biomechanics and Refractive Surgery*,
DOI 10.1007/978-1-4939-1767-9_4

The delayed postoperative response of the cornea is also of great interest. The mechanisms producing such responses are not well understood and may result from both cellular action and structural changes. The latter may be associated with weakening of the corneal integrity in response to damage mechanisms, wound healing processes, or changes in corneal thickness. Time-dependent or delayed regression of optical correction is a topic that is currently receiving some discussion in the literature. For example, some authors [2] have suggested that for higher levels of myopic correction, keratectasia might result. Those concerned over potential keratectasia for deeper ablation point to the evidence of refractive regression due to corneal central bulging over periods on the order of 3–12 months, although the mechanism for such a progressive change is not understood. This is a somewhat controversial issue, and a number of surgeons appear to be looking for a better appreciation of what might or might not be occurring. There appears to be no consensus on whether keratectasia is truly a complication of LASIK or not or whether it might be more indicated by keratoconus.

Since the physical mechanisms associated with possible time-dependent regression are far from understood, it does not seem feasible or useful to create models for these effects until we have more understanding. Nevertheless, a finite element model of the ablated cornea may be helpful in providing some insight into the nature of this problem. For example, if we created a very accurate model for deeper ablation, we could use the model to answer questions such as what changes in values of the elastic moduli would be necessary to cause significant and measurable keratectasia and what is the role of the ablation zone size, corneal thickness, IOP, limbal diameter, etc. The idea is that since we do not understand what tissue property changes are occurring postoperatively, we could use the finite element model to guide us in understanding what parameters might or might not be capable of creating keratectasia.

It is proposed to develop a finite element-based computer simulation tool for modeling the mechanical response of the cornea to excimer laser photoablation and to use it for parametric studies on laser surgery of the cornea.

This work has been performed in collaboration with Professor Peter Pinsky, from Division of Mechanics and Computation, Department of Mechanical Engineering, during my visit to Stanford University as visiting scholar. The work was funded by CONICET and Visx, Inc (Santa Clara, CA). This work was divided in two Phases (I and II).

Phase I was an initial effort to create the computational simulation framework and perform preliminary analyses of selected surgical procedures to verify the numerical model.

The broad objectives of the project are:

- To create and calibrate a general purpose finite element model for corneal tissue
- To apply the finite element model to simulation of myopic and hyperopic LASIK and investigate the role of the mechanical response of the tissue to these procedures

In the Phase II study, we have focused on the following primary tasks:

1. Develop a transversely isotropic constitutive model for the cornea including the nonlinear stiffening based on collagen stretching.
2. Parameter evaluation studies based on (1) cornea inflation experimental studies and (2) incisional surgery including ALK, RK, and LASIK.
3. Develop a hydration model for the cornea based on a biphasic theory.
4. Parameter identification and model validation based on data from in vivo profilometry of the LASIK procedure.
5. To investigate the mechanics of LASIK.

Two issues are crucial for reliable and accurate modeling of the cornea:

1. The mathematical representation of the mechanical properties of the cornea in the form of a general stress–strain relationship
2. Determination of the appropriate values for the model parameters

The mathematical modeling of the constitutive behavior is challenging because of the anisotropic and nonlinear nature of the stromal tissue. Determining the value of numerous properties is made difficult by the scarcity of data on in vivo mechanical behavior.

The modeling used in the Phase I study was based on the following three fundamental assumptions:

1. The corneal tissue is hyperelastic and isotropic. The hyperelastic assumption allows the characterization of the tissue in terms of a strain energy density that is a potential for the stress. The isotropic assumption states that material properties are the same in all directions.
2. The tissue can be modeled as a single-phase solid (elastic) material in which the fluid phase need not be explicitly modeled.
3. The nonlinearity in the tissue is expressed in terms of the strain invariants, and hence all strain components contribute.

There are indications that these assumptions are too restrictive and may be limiting for the subtle modeling needed for LASIK. In the Phase II study, we have revised and expanded the modeling capability to address all three of the above limitations. In particular, we have:

1. Developed a transversely isotropic finite deformation constitutive model.
2. Created a nonlinear theory that includes an exponential stiffness that is based directly on stretching of collagen fibers.
3. Developed a biphasic model for the cornea that models the cornea as having two interacting solid and fluid phases. For the fluid, we have assumed an inviscid fluid which contributes a pressure to the mixture and which is free to move through the solid skeleton.

1.1 Development of General Model for an Individual Lamella

Our approach is to first develop a model for a typical lamella and then create a cornea model by homogenizing (i.e., averaging) the lamella model through the stroma in an appropriate manner (Fig. 4.1). We start the lamella model by assuming that the collagen fibrils are oriented along the lamella with the characteristic direction indicated by a unit vector $\mathbf{a}$.

We then postulate that a *strain energy density* W for an individual lamella takes the form [4]

$$W(\mathbf{C}, \mathbf{a} \otimes \mathbf{a}) = W(Q \cdot \mathbf{C} \cdot Q^T, Q \cdot \mathbf{a} \otimes \mathbf{a} \cdot Q^T)$$

where $\mathbf{C}$ is the right Cauchy–Green deformation tensor, $\mathbf{a}$ is the orientation of the lamella (and also of the collagen fibrils within the lamella) relative to a fixed Cartesian coordinate frame, and Q is an arbitrary orthogonal transformation tensor. This implies that W is a function of five invariants:

$$
\begin{aligned}
I_1 &= \mathrm{tr}\mathbf{C} \\
I_2 &= \frac{1}{2}\left\{ (\mathrm{tr}\mathbf{C})^2 - \mathrm{tr}\mathbf{C}^2 \right\} \\
I_3 &= \det\mathbf{C} = J^2 \\
I_4 &= \mathbf{a} \cdot \mathbf{C} \cdot \mathbf{a} = \lambda^2 \\
I_5 &= \mathbf{a} \cdot \mathbf{C}^2 \cdot \mathbf{a}
\end{aligned}
$$

where λ is the stretch of collagen fibers oriented with direction $\mathbf{a}$.

The strain energy density is assumed to be additively decomposed into three parts:

1. The part W_T describes the isotropic ground substance.
2. The part W_L describes the collagen fibrils with orientation a.

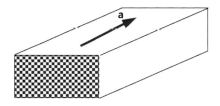

Fig. 4.1 Individual lamella showing orientation of the collagen fibrils

3. The part W_Q describes the fibril–fibril cross-linking and fibril–ground substance interaction.

We have postulated a model of the form:

$$W = W_T + W_L + W_Q \tag{4.1}$$

Where

$$
\begin{aligned}
W_T &= \frac{\mu_T}{2}(I_1 - 3) - \frac{\mu_T}{2}\ln I_3 + \frac{\lambda_T}{2}\left(\ln\sqrt{I_3}\right)^2 \\
W_L &= \frac{1}{4}\beta\left[\int e^\gamma(I_4 - 1)dI_4 - 1\right] + d(I_4 - 1) \\
W_C &= \frac{1}{4}\alpha(I_1 - 3)(I_4 - 3) + \frac{1}{2}(\mu_L - \mu_T)(I_5 - 1)
\end{aligned}
$$

and where λ_T, μ_T, μ_L, α, β, and d are constants. Only five are independent (see below), and values for these must be identified from appropriate experiments.

For hyperelasticity, the stress may be found from the gradient of the strain energy density with respect to its conjugate strain. This tells us that

$$\mathbf{S} = 2\frac{\partial W}{\partial \mathbf{C}} \tag{4.2}$$

where $\mathbf{S}$ is the second Piola–Kirchhoff stress, and $\mathbf{C}$ is (as above) the right Cauchy–Green deformation tensor. For our model, the stress in the lamina is found from

$$\mathbf{S} = 2\left(\frac{\partial W_T}{\partial \mathbf{C}} + \frac{\partial W_L}{\partial \mathbf{C}} + \frac{\partial W_C}{\partial \mathbf{C}}\right)$$

This provides us with a rather general and powerful model for a lamella.

1.2 Corneal Model with Rotational Averaging of Lamella

Since lamellae make large angles with adjacent overlying and underlying lamellae and since they have random orientation in the corneal plane, we introduce a rotational averaging (Fig. 4.2) of the energy density function of the form

$$W' = \frac{1}{\pi}\int_0^\pi \Phi(\mathbf{x}, \theta)W(\mathbf{a})d\theta$$

where each vector $\mathbf{a}$ provides the dependence on θ (in fact $\theta6 = \arctan(\alpha02/\alpha1)$), and $\Phi(\theta)$ is a weighting function of θ which can be used to describe nonuniform angular distribution of lamellae in different regions of the cornea (e.g., preferential

Fig. 4.2 Setup for angular averaging of lamella properties

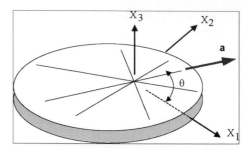

orientation at the limbus). Since the ground substance has been assumed isotropic, its contribution will be independent of the angular averaging. Accordingly, we set

$$W' = W_T + \frac{1}{\pi}\int_0^\pi \Phi(\mathbf{x},\theta)[W_L(\mathbf{a}) + W_L(\mathbf{a})]d\theta$$
$$= W_T + W'_L + W'_C$$

For uniform distribution of the fibrils, we will use

$$(\mathbf{x},\theta) = 1 \tag{4.3}$$

See [5] for nonuniform distribution of the fibrils.

The new constitutive equation for stress is now

$$\mathbf{S} = 2\left(\frac{\partial W_T}{\partial \mathbf{C}} + \frac{\partial W'_L}{\partial \mathbf{C}} + \frac{\partial W'_C}{\partial \mathbf{C}}\right)$$

The above theory has been implemented using the finite element method.

2 Calibration Studies for the Corneal Model

2.1 *Introduction*

We have used published experimental and clinical data as resources for identifying material parameter values as well as for verifying the model. The scope of this work is as follows:

1. ALK for hyperopia (Phases I and II)
2. Inflation tests on enucleated eyes (Phases I and II)
3. Normo-hydrated regional strain inflation experiments of Hjortdal
4. Radial keratotomy
5. VISX-sponsored profilometry study

We have found that the inflation tests of Hjortdal, controlling the hydration by using a solution of Dextran and keeping the corneal thickness constant during the experiment, provide a particularly useful data set and one that shows the considerable "stress stiffening" of the cornea. The profilometry study has promise but requires more work. In this section, we review results and conclusions from the calibration studies with the exception of profilometry which is discussed in Sect. 4.4.

2.2 Calibration with ALK-H and Inflation Tests

Our first attempt (Phase I) was to calibrate the model with a lamellar procedure, such as ALK for hyperopia, where the mechanical response is evident and desirable. A normal cornea is considered spherical with 7.8 mm of radius of curvature and 0.5 mm of apical thickness. From the nomograms of microkeratomes for ALK (see Manche et al. paper in JRS), it is found that a normal cornea with a flap thickness of 300 μm produces a 1 D of correction (steepening) and more for deeper laps.

Another calibration completed in Phase I was based on the membrane inflation tests of Bryant. We checked the material parameters obtained in this procedure by using the values in the ALK model to verify the microkeratome nomogram. We found that in two cases, with 300 and 375 μm flap thickness, there was agreement with the computed correction and the nomogram and thus consistency between the two data sets.

In PRK and LASIK, with these parameters, we found agreement for low values of correction. See Table 4.1 for a summary of results of ALK, PRK, and LASIK with the preliminary model calibrated with Bryant's inflation tests. Undercorrection of the attempted correction in diopters is shown in Tables 4.1 and 4.2.

These results suggest that improvement in the calibration of the model is needed. This has been a major focus of the Phase II study.

Table 4.1 Undercorrection of the attempted correction in diopters

ALK	
Attempted correction	Undercorrection
+1	0.2
+5	0.3

Table 4.2 Undercorrection of the attempted correction in diopters

	PRK	LASIK
Attempted correction	Undercorrection	Undercorrection
+2	0.7	1.0
+5	1.5	2.0

2.3   Normo-Hydrated Inflation Tests

The extensibility of 10 human corneas was evaluated in vitro by measuring central epithelial side strain induced by intraocular pressure loads ranging from 2 to 100 mmHg [3]. Corneal normo-hydration was attempted by immersing and perfusing the eyes with 8 % Dextran 500 in isotonic saline. The relation between corneal strain and intraocular pressure was found to be strongly nonlinear, showing a typical stress-stiffening behavior. This is strong evidence for the model approach described in Sect. 4.2. Compared with previous experiments performed with swollen corneas, the stiffness of the normo-hydrated human cornea was found to be higher. The complete description of the experimental technique can be found in [3].

In the model described in Sect. 4.2, the six parameters to be evaluated are $XT, fij, nL, a, [3,$ and 7. In practice, we have converted the first five of these constants to an equivalent set of constants denoted EA, Ej, vA, VT, and GA. This is done for convenience only since we can ascribe a more physical interpretation to this set of constants. Please see our technical paper for full details. The relationship between the sets is

$$
\begin{pmatrix} \lambda_T \\ \alpha \\ \beta \\ \mu_L \\ \mu_T \end{pmatrix} = \begin{pmatrix} k_x - G_T \\ G_T - k_x(1 - 2\nu A) \\ E_A + 4k_x\nu_A^2 + k_x + G_T - 4\nu_A k_x - 4G_A \\ G_A \\ G_T \end{pmatrix}
$$

$$
k_x = \frac{E_T}{2\left(1 - \nu_T - 2\nu_A^2\dfrac{E_T}{E_A}\right)}
$$

$$
G_T = \frac{E_T}{2(1 + \nu_T)}
$$

A series of studies were conducted to evaluate these constants resulting in the following estimates:

$$
\begin{aligned}
E_A &= 0.02 \quad \text{MPa} \\
E_T &= 0.02 \quad \text{MPa} \\
\nu_A &= 0.45 \\
\nu_T &= 0.45 \\
G_A &= 0.0039 \quad \text{MPa} \\
\gamma &= 270
\end{aligned}
$$

A plot of a typical experimentally measured IOP-strain curve versus the computed behavior is shown in Fig. 4.3.

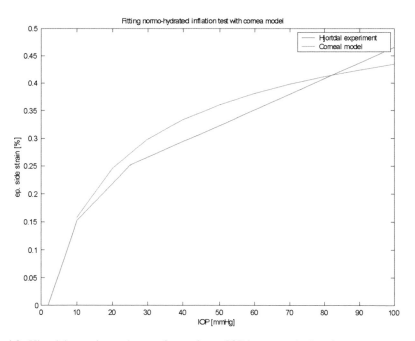

Fig. 4.3 Hjortdal experimental curve for strain vs. IOP in a norm-hydrated cornea compared to the computed curve with optimal material parameters

2.4   Simulation of RK and Comparison with Clinical Results

In addition to the regional strain patterns due to IOP, Hjortdal et al. studied the regional deformation pattern of the cornea after radial keratotomy [5]. The hydration was controlled in this experiment with a solution of 8 % Dextran T500 in 0.9 % NaCl for preserving the corneal thickness. In this experiment, four radial incisions were made with a double-edged diamond knife. The incision depth was set to 100 % of the central corneal thickness. The central optical zone was 3.5 mm. The incision was made from the center toward the periphery with subsequent redeepening. After the completion of the experiments, it was checked that the incisions penetrated to more than 90 % of the corneal thickness by histology.

The radial keratotomy induced 2.30 D of central flattening at an intraocular pressure of 2 mmHg. In the physiological pressure range, the central cornea flattened 0.05 D for each mmHg in intraocular pressure. The degree of central flattening correlated linearly with the amount of wound gape. Using the parameters fitted using the inflation test with an intact cornea, the central flattening at a physiological pressure of 16 mmHg was 3.9 D. The flattening measured by Hjortdal at 16 mmHg is 3.0 D. In general, we found a reasonable agreement between the RK data and the computed results confirming the parameter values. A typical result for the 3D RK model is shown in Fig. 4.4, where the contours indicate change in the z-contour.

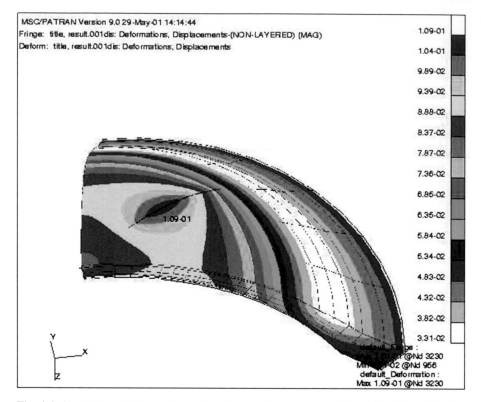

Fig. 4.4 Simulation of RK experiment based on model parameters obtained from intact inflation tests

3 Simulation of a Lamellar Surgery

Automated lamellar keratoplasty (ALK) can correct hyperopia by weakening the cornea with a deep lamellar resection. A thick section of the cornea is shaved by a microkeratome on a hinged flap. Then the corneal flap is replaced in its original position. Because the flap is thick, only a thin layer of posterior stroma remains. Intraocular pressure causes an iatrogenic corneal ectasia in the remaining stromal tissue under the flap. This causes a steepening of the central cornea, with reduction or elimination of the hyperopia. The safety and stability of the procedure is uncertain. A nomogram of ALK (automated lamellar keratoplasty) was used where a flap (similar to LASIK) is produced but deeper and then obtains a controlled "ectasia" to correct hyperopia.

We will compare the results of the model simulating ALK for hyperopia with a nomogram provided by the manufacturer of the microkeratome used in this procedure.

The geometry and mesh are shown in Fig. 4.5.

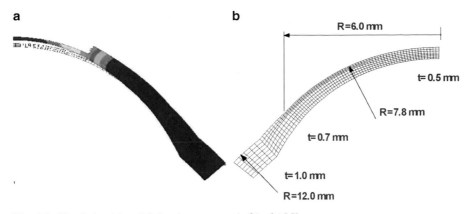

Fig. 4.5 Simulation (**a**) and finite elements mesh (**b**) of ALK surgery

ALK		
Table 4.3 Undercorrection of the attempted correction in diopters	Attempted correction	Undercorrection
	+1	0.2
	+5	0.3

From the nomogram, two extremes are simulated: using a flap of 300 and 375 μm. They produced a correction of +1 D and +5 D respectively, in a cornea of 500/μm. In Table 4.3, the undercorrection after simulation is shown for both flap thicknesses 300 (dashed lines) and 375 (solid lines). The agreement is quite good. Further analysis is necessary to account the behavior of the model for different central corneal thicknesses.

4 Finite Element Simulations of LASIK

By using the transversely isotropic model calibrated with normo-hydrated inflation test data (see Sect. 2.3), we modeled the LASIK procedure and compared the results to published clinical results. The results are summarized in this section.

4.1 Comparison of Attempted and Simulated Correction

In Fig. 4.6, we plot the attempted correction using Munnerlyn's equations and the achieved correction after the simulation of the LASIK procedure. The regression reported in LASIK after 1-year follow-up (poster in ARVO by [6]) indicates a

Fig. 4.6 Plot of attempted
and achieved correction
after simulation of LASIK
procedure

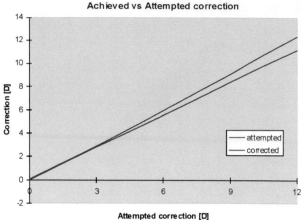

Table 4.4 Comparison of LASIK regression from clinical results [6] and simulation

	LASIK regression due to Velasco et al.		
	Low (−0.5 to −4 D)	Moderate (−4.25 to 8 D)	High (< −8.25 D)
Clinical results	−0.5	−0.84	−1.2
Simulation	−0.2	−0.5	−1.2 (for −12 D)

Fig. 4.7 Plot of
undercorrection in PRK
and LASIK

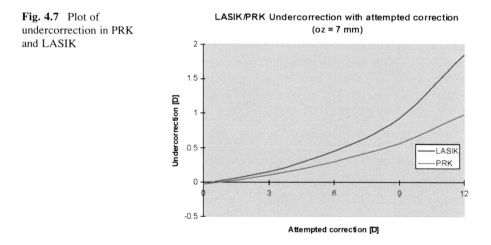

regression of −0.5, −0.84, and −1.2 D in refractive groups of −0.5 to 4, −4.25 to
8, and >−8.25 D, respectively. See Table 4.4 for comparison with simulation.

4.2   Undercorrection in PRK and LASIK

The undercorrection found for PRK and LASIK was different as shown in the
Fig. 4.7.

Fig. 4.8 Plot of undercorrection with the optical zone

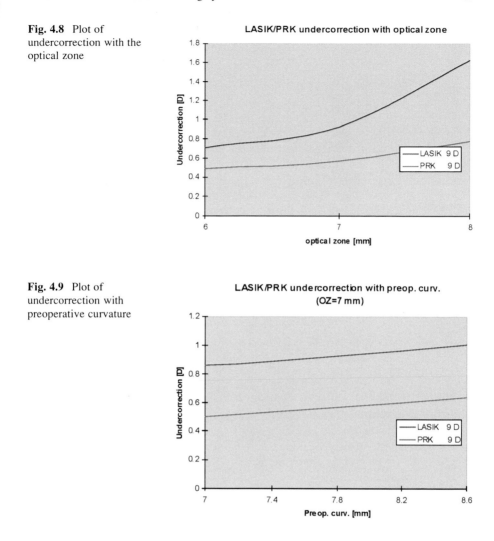

Fig. 4.9 Plot of undercorrection with preoperative curvature

4.3   *Undercorrection with the Optical Zone*

The sensitivity of undercorrection in LASIK due to varying the optical zone was important for higher diameters, as shown in Fig. 4.8.

4.4   *Undercorrection with the Preoperative Curvature*

Sensitivity to the preoperative curvature was small but increasing with the radius of curvature, as shown in Fig. 4.9.

4.5   Undercorrection with Ablation Depth and Optical Zone

Conclusions

In summary, we have accomplished the following tasks:

- Completed a model for transverse isotropy of the cornea based on its microstructural arrangement and features. This appears to be a useful model which has the correct convexity property and which will provide a basis for general cornea modeling as well as for extension to poroelasticity. The model has been implemented and tested in the special-purpose code FE-LASIK in both 3 D and axisymmetric versions using high-order elements (27-node hexahedrons in 3 D and 9-node quadrilaterals in axisymmetry).

- Completed further calibration based on experimental data for regional strains in normo-hydrated cornea inflation tests. These tests clearly indicate the nonlinear behavior of the tissue and the ability of the model to match the experiments. We used the calibrated model to simulate LASIK and appear to be obtaining reasonable results (although we have not yet introduced hydration effects in the LASIK modeling). We also verified the model parameters against studies of RK and achieved good correspondence of the computed results.

The delayed postoperative response of the cornea is also of great interest. The mechanisms producing such responses are not well understood and may result from both cellular action and structural changes. The latter may be associated with weakening of the corneal integrity in response to damage mechanisms, wound healing processes, or changes in corneal thickness. Time-dependent or delayed regression of optical correction is a topic that is currently receiving some discussion in the literature. For example, some authors [2] have suggested that for higher levels of myopic correction, keratectasia might result. Those concerned over potential keratectasia for deeper ablation point to the evidence of refractive regression due to corneal central bulging over periods in the order of 3 to 12 months, although the mechanism for such a progressive change is not understood. This is a somewhat controversial issue, and a number of surgeons appear to be looking for a better appreciation of what might or might not be occurring. There appears to be no consensus on whether keratectasia is truly a complication of LASIK or not or whether it might be more indicated by keratoconus.

References

1. K.D. Hanna, F.E. Jouve, G.O. Waring III, Preliminary computer simulation of the effects of radial keratotomy. Arch. Ophthalmol. **107**, 911–918 (1989)
2. T. Seiler, M. Matallana, S. Sendler, T. Bende, Does Bowman's layer determine the biomechanical properties of the cornea? Refract. Corneal. Surg. **8**(2), 139–142 (1992)
3. J.O. Hjortdal, N. Ehlers, Extensibility of the normo-hydrated human cornea. Acta Ophthalmol. Scand. **73**(1), 12–17 (1995)
4. A.J.M. Spencer, Constitutive theory for strongly anisotropic solids, in *Continuum Theory of the Mechanics of Fibre-Reinforced Composites* (Springer, Vienna, 1984), pp. 1–32
5. P.M. Pinsky, D. van der Heide, D. Chernyak, Computational modeling of mechanical anisotropy in the cornea and sclera. J. Cataract Refract. Surg. **31**(1), 136–145 (2005)
6. R. Velasco et al., Regression in LASIK with the Visx star excimer laser: one year follow up. Invest. Ophthalmol. Vis. Sci. **42**(4) (2001)

Chapter 5
Biomechanics of Additive Surgery: Intracorneal Rings

Fabio A. Guarnieri, Paulo Ferrara, and Leonardo Torquetti

1 Introduction

The aim of supervision relies on a thorough understanding of corneal biomechanics in order to predict refractive surgery outcome. The study of changes in stress and elasticity after corneal reshaping by additive or subtractive surgical techniques are very important in order to obtain reliable procedures.

Incisional procedures, as radial and astigmatic keratotomy, were developed empirically without detailed knowledge of corneal biomechanics. In PRK and LASIK, the cornea was considered as a piece of plastic, and the Munnerlyn equation was used to account the refractive outcome of the excimer laser. In order to obtain accuracy, predictability, and reproducibility to these procedures, regression analysis and empirical adjustments were introduced. But they are still problems with outliers like overcorrection, undercorrection, and ectasia. The attempt to correct higher myopes in lamellar procedures introduces the concept of biomechanical effects [Seiler]. Corneal biomechanical modelling helped to understand these effects [1].

F.A. Guarnieri, Ph.D. (✉)
Department of Bioengineering, Centro de Investigacion de Métodos Computacionales (CIMEC), Predio CONICET-Santa Fe, Colectora Ruta Nac 168, Km 472,
Paraje El Pozo, 3000 Santa Fe, Argentina
e-mail: aguarni@santafe-conicet.gov.ar

P. Ferrara, M.D., Ph.D.
Paulo Ferrara Eye Clinic, Keratoconus Unit, AV Contorno, 4747—Suite 615,
B. Serra, Belo Horizonte, MG 30110-090, Brazil
e-mail: pferrara@ferra8raring.com.br

L. Torquetti, M.D., Ph.D.
Center for Excellence in Ophthalmology, Anterior Segment, RUA Capitão Teixeira, 415,
B. Nossa Senhora das Graças, Pará de Minas, MG 35660-051, Brazil
e-mail: leonardo@ceoclinica.med.br

© Springer Science+Business Media New York 2015
F.A. Guarnieri (ed.), *Corneal Biomechanics and Refractive Surgery*,
DOI 10.1007/978-1-4939-1767-9_5

As in RK and AK, ICRS refractive outcome relies directly on corneal biomechanics. The concept of a ring-shaped device that could be introduced into the cornea through a single, peripheral, radial incision originated with Reynolds in 1978. This implant would alter the anterior corneal curvature by expansion of the device's diameter resulting in flattening (myopic correction) or by constriction to steepen the cornea (hyperopic correction).

The insertion of segments without expansion also resulted in corneal flattening. Silvestrini [2] proposed the "arc shortening theory" based on the tissue separation by the inserts producing a flattening in the anterior corneal surface. This mechanism was described thoroughly by Pinsky et al. using a corneal model by the finite element method [3]. While the Silvestrini mathematical model defined a linear relationship between ring thickness and flattening, Pinsky model allows predicting effect variations in physical and surgical parameters as thickness, width, diameter, cone angle, arc length, and materials. This model is used to predict different designs for myopia, astigmatism, and hyperopia.

Further modeling of the cornea has been developed in order to account its material nonlinearity, viscoelasticity, and anisotropy [1, 4]. This model has been used to simulate the behavior of the Ferrara ring segments in astigmatic and further in keratoconic eyes. The mechanical behavior of this implant is different since its triangular cross section combined with its nonconformal curvature to the curve of the cornea alters differently the anterior corneal surface. Moreover, in keratoconus, the corneal biomechanics is altered, and both geometrical and material changes should be accounted in order to have reliable and predictable results in ICRS surgery.

In this chapter corneal biomechanics and modelling of Ferrara ring implants in astigmatic and keratoconic corneas will be described.

2   Ferrara Rings and Keratoconus

Keratoconus is a corneal ectatic disease characterized by noninflammatory progressive thinning of unknown cause in which the cornea assumes a conical shape. Intracorneal ring segments have been used to correct ectatic corneal diseases in order to reduce the corneal steepening, reduce the irregular astigmatism, and improve the visual acuity [5–11]. Besides, the ring is a surgical alternative to at least delay, if not eliminate, the need of lamellar or penetrating keratoplasty.

The Ferrara ring segments are made of PMMA Perspex CQ acrylic segments. They vary in thickness and are available in 0.15, 0.20, 0.25, and 0.30 mm. The segment cross section is triangular, and the base for every thickness and diameter is 0.60 mm. The segments have 90°, 120°, 160°, or 210° of arc.

Many studies have demonstrated the efficacy of intrastromal rings to treat many corneal conditions as keratoconus [5–11], post-LASIK corneal ectasia [12], post-radial keratotomy ectasia [13], astigmatism [14], and myopia [15–18]. The changes in corneal structure induced by additive technologies can be roughly predicted by the Barraquer's thickness law; that is, when material is added to the periphery of the cornea or an equal amount of material is removed from the central area, a flattening effect is achieved. The corrective result varies in direct proportion to the thickness of the implant and in inverse proportion to its diameter. The thicker and smaller the diameter of the device, the higher the corrective result [19].

Preliminary investigations have demonstrated that intracorneal rings are effective in the treatment of astigmatism and myopia with astigmatism [19], with preservation of BSCVA and stable results over time [20]. The objective of the addictive technology is to reinforce the cornea, decrease the corneal irregularity, and provide an improvement of the visual acuity in affected patients.

The research about the Ferrara ring began in 1985. In 1986, we (P.F.) realized it was necessary a big hole in the center of the lens to keep the implant in place, which resulted in an annular prostheses. Since then we started trying several annular shapes and diameters and from these researches we concluded that the best project is the one we are using nowadays, made of PMMA, with a total diameter of 5.0 mm, arch length ranging from 90° to 210°, and thickness ranging from 100 to 400 microns.

The rings were implanted in rabbit eyes, through a free-hand dissection technique, at 50 % depth of measured central corneal thickness. The eyes were examined for 12 months, and the animals were sacrificed so that their eyes could be submitted to histopathological exams. The histopathological results revealed excellent tolerance of the cornea to the prostheses since there were only slight inflammatory reactions surrounding the implant and no evidence of extrusion.

The techniques traditionally used for the implant of corneal prostheses, free-hand dissection, and keratectomy with a microkeratome showed some negative points, such as interface deposits, delay in refractive stability, besides the high costs of the microkeratomes and slow learning curves.

In order to improve the ring implantation technique, reducing its complications and making it accessible to a large number of anterior segment surgeons, we (P.F.) developed in 1994 a stromal tunnel and ring implantation technique, which completely eliminates the disadvantages of the conventional techniques.

In 1995 we (P.F.) implanted the first patient who had undergone penetrating keratoplasty and radial keratotomy (Fig. 5.1). This patient was forwarded to the Cornea Service at Hospital Sao Geraldo in UFMG (Federal University of Minas Gerais) for a new transplantation. We decided, with formal authorization of the

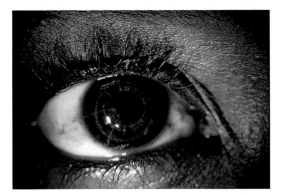

Fig. 5.1 First patient operated with the Ferrara ring (postkeratoplasty high astigmatism)

Fig. 5.2 Ferrara ring
implanted in a patient with
keratoconus

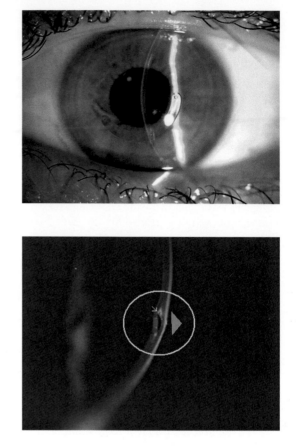

Fig. 5.3 Flat basis (*arrow*)
of the Ferrara ring

patient, to test the ring before performing the penetrating keratoplasty. The result
was satisfactory, yielding ametropia correction and perfect corneal tolerance to the
orthesis. After a 6-year follow-up, the patient has good uncorrected and corrected
visual acuity, the shape is more regular, and the refraction is stable.

The excellent tolerance to the implant by the transplanted cornea gave us the
necessary confidence to apply the technique in keratoconic corneas. Therefore, we
decided, in 1996, to implant the rings in patients intolerant to contact lenses that's
had the penetrating keratoplasty indicated (Fig. 5.2).

2.1   The Ferrara Ring Characteristics

The Ferrara ring has the following characteristics (Fig. 5.3):

– Total diameter (external) of 5.6 mm
– Triangular section
– 600-micron base

- Variable thickness
- One or two 1,600 segments
- One orifice in each extremity
- Yellow PMMA

2.2   How the Ferrara Ring Works

The corneal ring complies with Barraquer and Blavatskaya postulates, according to those an addition in the cornea periphery results in its flattening, and the ring diameter determines how much the cornea will be flattened. Thus, the more tissue is added (increasing ring thickness), and the smaller the diameter, the greater will be the myopia correction obtained [20, 21].

Our study resulted in the additional observations presented below:

- Central and peripheral flattening of the cornea, preserving its asphericity.
- Decrease in the anterior chamber depth as shown in ultrasonic biomicroscopy.
- Regularization of the corneal surface through a tilting movement caused by the flatness in the surface of the ring basis, making the cornea flattened at the areas corresponding to the segments extremities and making it curve at the ring's body area.
- Interruption or at least delay of keratoconus evolution, diminishing opacity on the cone apex, and reduction of related symptoms as itching, photophobia, and pain and/or ocular discomfort.
- Lack of correspondence between visual acuity uncorrected after surgery and residual ametropia. Sometimes it can be observed with good vision coexisting with high residual refractive errors.
- The prisma effect generated by the triangular section eliminates the halos and glare, which could result from the small diameter of the orthesis.
- The yellow filter introduced in the plastic avoids the UV light to go into the eye reducing thus the halos and reflections at night.

2.3   Indications

The main indication for the Ferrara ring implantation is the keratoconus. In patients with keratoconus the Ferrara ring is indicated when there is evidence of progressive worsening of the disease, with gradual decrease of uncorrected visual acuity (UCVA) and best-corrected visual acuity (BCVA) and progressive corneal steepening. In patients with unsatisfactory BCVA with glasses and intolerance to contact lenses the Ferrara ring implantation is also indicated.

Table 5.1 Ferrara ring indications

1.	Keratoconus
2.	High irregular astigmatisms after penetrating or lamellar keratoplasty
3.	Irregular astigmatisms after radial keratotomy
4.	Pellucid marginal degeneration
5.	Corneal ectasia after excimer laser

Table 5.2 Ferrara ring contraindications

1.	Very advanced keratoconus with curvatures over 75 diopters and significant apical opacity and scarring
2.	Hydropsis
3.	Thin corneas, with thickness below 300 microns in the ring track
4.	Patients with intense atopia (these should be treated before the implant)
5.	Any ongoing infectious process, local or systemic

In post-LASIK corneal ectasia the Ferrara ring implantation is indicated when there is worsening of the condition. The main indications for the Ferrara ring implantation are listed in the Table 5.1.

2.4 Contraindications

The main contraindications for Ferrara ring implantation is the presence of apical opacities in very advanced keratoconus, usually with K readings above 75 D. The postoperative results in these cases are usually poor, and the best treatment for these cases is the lamellar or penetrating keratoplasty. The main contraindications for the Ferrara ring implantation are listed in the Table 5.2.

2.5 Nomogram

The nomogram has evolved as the knowledge about the predictability of results has grown. Initially, surgeons implanted a pair of symmetrical segments in every case. The incision was always placed on the steep meridian to take advantage of the coupling effect achieved by the rings.

First, only the grade of keratoconus was considered for the ring selection, which means that in keratoconus grade I, the more suitable Ferrara ring for implantation was that of 150 μm and in the keratoconus grade IV, the more appropriate ring was of 350 μm (Table 5.3). However, some cases of extrusion could be observed; as in keratoconus grade IV, the cornea usually is very thin and the thick ring segment sometimes was not properly fitted into the corneal stroma.

Table 5.3 Dr. Paulo Ferrara original (first generation) nomogram

Diameter 5.00 mm	Thickness diopters to be corrected
Frustre 0.150 mm	−2.00 to −4.00
Cone I 0.200 mm	−4.25 to −6.00
Cone II 0.250 mm	−6.25 to −8.00
Cone III 0.300 mm	−8.25 to −10.00
Cone IV 0.350 mm	−10.25 to −12.00

Map	Distribution of Ectasia	Description
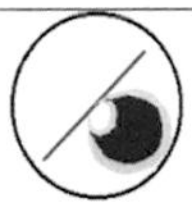	**0 % / 100%**	All the ectatic area is located at one side of the cornea
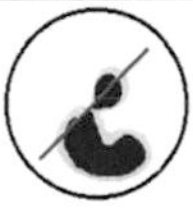	**25 % / 75%**	75% of the ectatic area is located at one side of the cornea
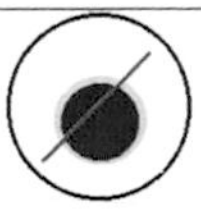	**33 % / 66%**	66% of the ectatic area is located at one side of the cornea
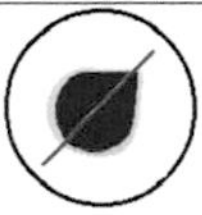	**50 % / 50%**	The ectatic area is symmetrically distributed on the cornea

Fig. 5.4 Distribution of the area of corneal ectasia. The ectatic area is symmetrically distributed on the cornea

The second generation of the nomogram considered the refraction for the ring selection, besides the distribution of the ectatic area on the cornea. Therefore, as the spherical equivalent increased, the selected ring thickness also increased. However, in many keratoconus cases the myopia and astigmatism could not be caused by the ectasia itself but by an increase in the axial length of the eye (axial myopia). In these cases, a hypercorrection by implanting a thick ring segment in a keratoconus in which a thinner segment was indicated was observed.

In the third and actual generation of the Ferrara ring nomogram, the ring selection depends on the type of keratoconus, its location in the cornea (Fig. 5.4), corneal asphericity (Q), topographic astigmatism (Tables 5.4, 5.5, and 5.6), and pachymetry [22–24].

For symmetric bow tie patterns of keratoconus, two equal segments are selected. For nipple cones, a single 210 μm segment is chosen based on the nomogram (Table 5.7). For peripheral cones, the most common form type, asymmetrical

Table 5.4 Segment thickness choice in symmetric bow tie keratoconus

Topographic astigmatism (D)	Segment thickness
<1.00	150/150
1.25–2.00	200/200
2.25–3.00	250/250
>3.25	300/300

Table 5.5 Asymmetrical segment thickness choice in sag cones with 0/100 and 25/75 % of asymmetry index (Fig. 5.1)

Topographic astigmatism (D)	Segment thickness
<1.00	None/150
1.25–2.00	None/200
2.25–3.00	None/250
3.25–4.00	None/300
4.25–5.00	150/250
6.25–6.00	200/300

Table 5.6 Asymmetrical segment thickness choice in sag cones with 0/100 and 33/66 % of asymmetry index (Fig. 5.1)

Topographic astigmatism (D)	Segment thickness
<1.00	None/150
1.25–2.00	150/200
2.25–3.00	200/250
3.25–4.00	250/300

Table 5.7 Segment thickness choice in nipple cones (210/m ring)

Spherical equivalent (D)	Segment thickness
Up to 2.00	150
2.25–4.00	200
4.25–6.00	250
>6.25	300

Table 5.8 Ferrara ring nomogram: step by step

1.	Define the keratoconus type: sag, bow tie or nipple
2.	Distribution of the ectatic area in the cornea: 0/100, 25/75, 50/50, and 33/66
3.	Corneal asphericity (Q)
4.	Topographic astigmatism
5.	Pachymetry at incision site and ring track

segments are selected. It is important to emphasize that the ring segment thickness cannot exceed 50 % of the thickness of the cornea on the track of the ring.

The first step in ring selection is to define the type of keratoconus of the patient: sag, bow tie, or nipple. After, it is determined the distribution of the keratoconus in the cornea: central (nipple and bow tie) or paracentral (asymmetric) (0/100, 25/75, and 33/66; Fig. 5.2). The next step is to evaluate the preoperative corneal asphericity value (Q), which is desirable but not indispensable, as most corneal topographers do not show this data. However, preliminary data shows that the corneal asphericity may be linked to the quality of vision; therefore, when possible, this data should be obtained by corneal topographers (Orbscan and Pentacam) to achieve the best possible visual results. We have described (unpublished study) that for each ring segment there is a correspondent Q value reduction (Fig. 5.4). A target postoperative Q value closest possible of −0.23 is the goal after Ferrara ring implantation.

The topographic astigmatism defines the thickness of the rings to be implanted (Tables 5.4, 5.5, and 5.6). The only type of keratoconus that does not depend on the topographic astigmatism for ring selection is the nipple conus. In this case the spherical equivalent defines the thickness of the ring to be implanted, which should be a 210-arc ring, which is indicated exclusively for this type of keratoconus [20].

The pachymetry at the incision site (steep axis of the cornea) must be determined. The incision depth must be 80 % of the cornea thickness at the incision site. The pachymetry should be measured in all ring tracks to avoid superficial rings, which could lead to future extrusion.

2.6 Surgical Technique

2.6.1 Manual Technique

The surgery is performed under topical anesthesia after miosis achieved with 2 % pilocarpine. An eyelid speculum is used to expose the eye, and a 2.5 % povidone–iodine eyedrops is instilled into the cornea and conjunctival cul-de-sac. The visual axis is marked by pressing the Sinskey hook on the central corneal epithelium while asking the patient to fixate on the corneal light reflex of the microscope light. Using a marker tinted with gentian-violet, a 5.0 mm optical zone and incision site are aligned to the desired axis in which the incision will be made. This site can be the steepest topographic axis of the cornea (in case of implantation of two segments) or 900 (in case of implantation of only one segment—one of the tips of the ring must be located on the steepest axis).

The depth of a 1.0 mm square diamond blade is set at 80 % of corneal thickness at the incision site, and this blade is used to make the incision. Using a "stromal spreader," a pocket is formed in each side of the incision. Two (clockwise and counterclockwise) 2,700 semicircular dissecting spatulas are consecutively inserted through the incision and gently pushed with some, quick, rotary "back and forth" tunneling movements. Following channel creation, the ring segments are inserted using a modified McPherson forceps. The rings are properly positioned with the aid of a Sinskey hook.

2.6.2   Femtosecond Laser Technique

The femtosecond laser (IntraLase Corp.) has been recently introduced in clinical practice whose surgical effect via photodisruption can be used as an alternative to traditional mechanical techniques. Several recent papers [25–28] have reported its efficacy and safety for tunnel creation and intrastromal rings implantation. The femtosecond laser can easily and quickly create a predetermined depth and channel size.

There is controversy over channel size nomograms with the technique. Some authors conclude that more effects can be achieved by making the stromal channels narrower than the ring size, leading to faster visual results [29].

The use of the femtosecond laser in corneal tunnel creation made the procedure faster, easier (especially for inexperienced surgeons), and more comfortable for the patient. However, the main advantage of IntraLase-assisted channel creation over the mechanical technique seems to be the precise depth of implantation. The only advantage of this technique is the cost of the equipment, which is high.

The technique: tunnel depth is set at 80 % of the thinnest corneal thickness on the tunnel location in the femtosecond laser. Special attention must be given in centralizing the disposable suction ring to mark the central point to minimize decentration. The channel's inner diameter is set to 4.4 mm, the outer diameter 5.6 mm, the entry cut thickness is 1 m (at the steepest topographic axis), the ring energy used for channel creation is 1.30j, and the entry cut energy is 1.30j. Channel creation timing with the femtosecond laser is 15 s. The intracorneal ring segments are implanted immediately after channel creation before the disappearance of the bubbles, which reveals the exact tunnel location. The segments are placed in the final position with a Sinskey hook through a dialing hole at both ends of the segment.

The postoperative regimen, for both techniques, consists of moxiloxacin 0.5 % (*Vigamox®*, *Alcon*, USA) and dexamethasone 0.1 % (Maxidex®, Alcon, USA) eyedrops four times daily for two weeks. The patients were instructed to avoid rubbing the eye and to use preservative-free artificial tears frequently—Polyethylene Glycol 400 0.4 % (Oftane®, Alcon, USA).

2.7   Clinical Results: Long-Term Follow-Up in Keratoconus [21]

We retrospectively reviewed patient records of 94 eyes of 76 patients, which were consecutively operated (Ferrara ring implantation). There were 33 females and 61 males. The average age of the patients was 28.1 years. All procedures were performed by the same surgeon (PF), between June of 1996 and September of 2007. Patients included in the study presented clear cornea and a minimal corneal thickness of 300 μm at the ring track. Patients were intolerant to contact lens and/or showed progression of the ectasia.

Fifty-eight subjects underwent to a single eye treatment, whereas 18 subjects had both eye treated. Seventy-three eyes had a 2-year follow-up, 66 eyes had a 3-year follow-up, 48 eyes had a 4-year follow-up, and 34 eyes had a 5-year follow-up. All patients completed at least a 2-year follow-up. No intraoperative complications occurred during the procedures. All patients returned for ocular examination on day one, 1 week, and a month after the surgery and then 3, 6, and 12 months. Thereafter, the following eye examinations occurred yearly.

Preoperative and postoperative UCVA, BSCVA, and keratometry data were collected from all patients. The mean UCVA at the preoperative period was 0.12, and the mean BSCVA was 0.41. At the first month, the mean UCVA improved to 0.25, and the mean BSCVA improved to 0.56. At the second-year follow-up, the mean UCVA improved from 0.12 preoperatively to 0.29. At the third-year follow-up, the mean UCVA improved to 0.34; at the fourth-year follow-up, the mean UCVA improved to 0.42; and at the fifth-year follow-up, the mean UCVA decreased to 0.31 postoperatively. The mean BSCVA, at the 1st month, improved to 0.56. At the second-year follow-up, the mean BSCVA improved from 0.41 preoperatively to 0.68. At the third-year follow-up, the mean BSCVA decreased to 0.63; at the fourth-year follow-up, the mean BSCVA improved to 0.65; and at the fifth-year follow-up, the mean BSCVA decreased to 0.59 postoperatively (Fig. 5.5).

Mean keratometry decreased significantly from the preoperative to the last post-operative follow-up. Preoperative mean keratometry was 50.36, which de creases to 47.29 at 1st month postoperative follow-up. The mean keratometry follow-up along the second to fifth years was 45.96, 45.83, 46.44, and 46.24, respectively. The topography showed a decrease in the corneal steepening at the postoperative period, flattening of the central cornea, and displacement of the central cornea.

As showed in previous studies the intrastromal ring flattens the cornea and keeps this effect for a long period of time. There is no significant re-steepening of the cornea over time.

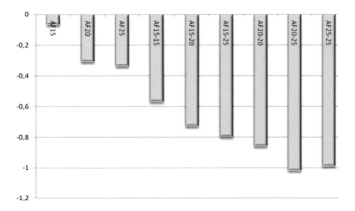

Fig. 5.5 Q (asphericity) variation according to ring thickness

The present study showed that the Ferrara ring, despite the small sample of patients, can be a valuable tool to provide topographic and visual stability, delay the progression of keratoconus, and postpone a corneal grafting surgery to a more physiological position.

2.8 Clinical Results: The 210 Ferrara Ring [20]

The 210° of arc Ferrara intrastromal ring (210-FICR), which is a novel FICR, has three major advantages over the conventional ring: (1) minimal astigmatic induction, (2) corneal flattening, and (3) implantation of a single segment. This ring is especially useful for the nipple type of keratoconus. The 210-FICR is an efficient method for keratoconus correction, significantly decreasing the keratometric values and spherical equivalent and improving UCVA and BCVA.

We retrospectively reviewed patient records of 80 eyes of 76 patients, which were consecutively operated, in which the 210-FICR was implanted. Statistical analysis included preoperative and postoperative uncorrected visual acuity (UCVA), best-corrected visual acuity (BCVA), spherical equivalent, and keratometry.

The mean follow-up time was 6.65 months. The mean UCVA increased from 20/350 to 20/136 ($p = 0.001$). The mean BCVA increased from 20/125 to 20/55 ($p = 0.0001$). The mean preoperative spherical equivalent decreased from -5.22 D, preoperative, to -2.26 D ($p = 0.050$), postoperative.

Corneal tomography (Pentacam^) showed corneal flattening in all eyes.

The mean K1 decreased from 51.49 D to 47.40 D ($p = 0.00014$), and the mean K2 decreased from 54.33 D to 49.14 D ($p = 0.00022$). The mean keratometric astigmatism decreased from 3.65 D (preoperative) to 2.69 D (postoperative) ($p = 0.0001$).

2.9 Clinical Results: Post-Refractive Surgery Corneal Ectasia [30]

Twenty-five eyes of 20 patients with corneal ectasia (13 males [15 eyes] and 7 females [10 eyes]) who underwent Ferrara intracorneal ring segments (ICRS) implantation were included in this study.

The mean follow-up time was 39.8 ± 21.1 months (Table 5.1). All patients were implanted only one segment of ICRS in 18 eyes and the 210° of arc (210—ICRS) ring was implanted in 7 eyes.

The mean UDVA increased from 20/185 to 20/66 ($p = 0.005$). The mean CDVA increased from 20/125 to 20/40 ($p = 0.008$) (Fig. 5.4). The mean asphericity values decreased from -0.95, preoperatively, to -0.23 ($p = 0.006$), postoperatively.

The mean pachymetry at the apex of the cornea increased from (mean) 457.7 ± 48.7^m (range 361–542) to 466.2 ± 49.8^m (range 381–559) ($p = 0.025$), and the pachymetry at thinnest point of the cornea increased from 436.3 ± 46.2^m (range 348–533) to 453.9 ± 49.3^m (range 370–548) ($p = 0.000$). A significant reduction in keratometric values was found at the last follow-up examination; mean preoperative keratometry was decreased from 45.41 ± 5.63 D (range 37.3–55.5) and changed significantly to 42.88 ± 4.44D (range 31.2–54.1) ($p = 0.000$) (Fig. 5.5).

Our postoperative results show a significant improvement in UDVA and CDVA. Moreover, there was significant increase in corneal thickness. This can be explained by a theoretically cornea collagen remodeling induced by the implantation of ICRS.

We found a significant decrease in asphericity values after implantation of ICRS in this study. Interestingly, the mean postoperative value was −0.23, which is considered the "normal" value for the general population. This value means that the normal physiologic asphericity of the cornea shows a significant individual variation ranging from mild oblate to moderate prolate. In an unpublished study, where we evaluated the corneal asphericity changes induced by the ICRS in keratoconus, we found that the Ferrara intrastromal ring implantation significantly reduced the mean corneal asphericity from −0.85 to −0.32. It is well known that most corneas after ablation laser procedures tend to become oblate, and when the ectasia develops, these corneas usually become prolate. However, the excess of prolatism usually found in keratoconus (primary) is usually of a much larger amount that one found in post-refractive surgery ectasia. That is the probable reason the Q value after FICR becomes much closer to "normal" values than when the ring is used for keratoconus. As the asphericity is one of the markers of visual quality, turning it "normal" can be a predictor of improvement of visual quality.

The keratometry values reduced significantly in all eyes. It can be realized that the mean preoperative values are usually lower than the ones found in keratoconus (primary). This can be explained somewhat by the corneal flattening induced by the refractive procedure, usually in an optic zone of greater extent than the location of the ectasia.

Most of the implanted ICRS were 160-FICR, the "conventional" ring. The remainder of the eyes received the 210-ICRS. The latter is usually reserved for central cones of nipple type. Some ectasia assumes the same topographical pattern of nipple cones, in which we usually use the 210-FICR with excellent results [17]. This ring is reserved for cases with low astigmatism, in which we desire to flatten the cornea with minimal astigmatic induction.

The potential advantages of ICRS implantation over keratoplasty in eyes with post-LASIK ectasia are many. First, it avoids further laser treatment, eliminating central corneal wound healing. This leaves the optical center of the cornea untouched, enhancing the refractive outcome. Second, the technique is reversible in cases of unsatisfactory refractive or clinical outcomes, and minimal postoperative care is required. Third, adjustment can be performed using thinner or thicker rings. In cases of unexpected corneal shape changes, 1 segment can be removed or exchanged. Fourth, it avoids the complications of intraocular surgery.

2.10   Clinical Results: Endothelium Evaluation [31]

We retrospectively reviewed patient records of 102 eyes of 81 patients, which were followed for a period of at least 1 year (mean follow-up, 45.7 months; SD, 16.4 months; range, 13–71 months). All patients had the diagnosis of keratoconus, post-LASIK ectasia, or pellucid degeneration. Statistical analysis included preoperative and postoperative keratometry and endothelial characteristics (cell count, average cell size, and coefficient of variation).

All patients completed at least 1 year of follow-up (range 13–71 months). Mean age was 30.5 ± 8 years. The mean cell count decreased from (mean $\pm$ SD) $2,714 \pm 372$ to $2,562 \pm 406$ cells/mm^2 ($p < 0.001$). The calculated exponential cell loss rate over the mean interval follow-up (4 years) was 1.4 % per year. The average cell size increased from (mean $\pm$ SD) 375 ± 56 μ^2 to $399 \pm 61/2$ ($p < 0.001$). The coefficient of variation increased from (mean $\pm$ SD) 0.22 ± 0.075 to 0.26 ± 0.010 ($p = 0.001$). All corneas remained clear during the follow-up period.

The mean maximum cell size increased from (mean $\pm$ SD) 529 ± 116 to 639 ± 225 μ^2 ($p < 0.001$). The mean minimum cell size varied from (mean $\pm$ SD) 225 ± 36 to 226 ± 54 μ^2 ($p = 0.936$).

There was significant corneal flattening as showed by keratometry changes. The mean K decreased from 47.70 ± 2.29 (range 43.70–53.80) to 44.86 ± 2.02 (range 41.20–51.20) ($p = 0.0001$).

In our study we found a 1.4 % loss of endothelial cells per year. Considering that most of the studied patients were young, the rate of endothelial cell loss was slightly higher than in normal eyes (1.1 %). Moreover, there is no study in the current literature that shows the profile of the "normal" endothelial loss in keratoconus corneas, which could be higher than in normal corneas. The only report in the literature regarding the endothelium profile of keratoconus is non-prospective and studied only 12 eyes [32].

Endothelial cell loss after penetrating keratoplasty is known to be an ongoing process even years after surgery. It is well known that the cell loss is higher in the early time course after surgery and decreases 3–5 years after surgery. There is a great variation of rates of cell loss after PK, ranging from 4.2 [33] to 9.4 % [34] per year, at the long-term follow-up. Even after DALK, which is a surgical technique that spares the receptor endothelium, cell loss has been reported [19]. In one study, a decrease in average endothelial cell count from preoperative of approximately 200 cells/mm^2 was observed during the first 12 months after surgery.

The only study [35], which assessed the endothelial after intrastromal rings (Intacs, Addition Technology Inc) implantation reported that at 24 months after surgery, all corneal regions had a slight decrease in cell density. In all eyes, the mean central and peripheral endothelial cell counts remained above 2,495 cells/mm^2. Our results are similar; we obtained a higher average postoperative cell count (2,562 cells/mm^2), and we had a longer follow-up (4 years).

Woolensak et al. [36] in a collagen cross-linking study in keratoconus showed that the corneal transparency and the endothelial cell density ($p = 0.45$) remained unchanged. The follow-up was 23 months, and the sample was only 23 eyes. The same author, in an experimental study in rabbits [27], showed that riboflavin-UVA treatment should be safe as long as the dose is less than the endothelial cytotoxic dose of 0.65 J/cm^2. In human corneas the endothelial cytotoxic UVA dose is reached in corneas thinner than 400, which is not uncommon in keratoconus patients. Moreover, the data obtained from normal corneas of rabbit cannot be extrapolated to human keratoconic corneas, which can have a different metabolism and response to cross-linking. The study has a limitation of measuring the endothelial toxicity only at 4 and 24 h after treatment. The long-term endothelial cytotoxicity was not evaluated by the study.

Our study suggests that some endothelial changes occur after Ferrara ring implantation. However, these changes are minimal and nonclinically significant, since the endothelial cell loss rate is not much higher than the normally expected for normal corneas. In contrast, the long-term endothelial cell loss after other therapies for keratoconus is much higher (as in PK, or even DALK, in which the receptor endothelium is spared) or unknown (as in cross-linking).

2.11 Contact Lens Wear After Ferrara Ring Implantation

Contact lens wear in keratoconus patients can be considerably facilitated after Ferrara ring implantation. Once there is corneal surface regularization with reduction of the excess of prolatism, the majority of patients can be well fitted with contact lens after the surgery.

The contact lens trial must be done only after 3 months of surgery, which is the period required for keratometry and refraction stabilization. It is very common that patients that usually were intolerant to rigid gas-permeable contact lens in the preoperative period become tolerant after the surgery. Moreover, there is very good stability of the contact lenses after the surgery, with "losses of lenses" caused by instability (a common complaint before the surgery) not occurring anymore.

2.12 Complications

The incidence of complications after the learning curve is very low. Postoperative complications can be related to (1) the surgical technique, (2) the nomogram, and (3) the ring itself. The complications related to the surgical technique are extrusion (due to a shallow tunnel), infection, bad centration of the segment (wrong placement of the ring), migration, and misplacement or asymmetry of the segments.

The complications related to the nomogram are linked to the corneal biomechanics and can be (1) overcorrection and (2) undercorrection. Although the predictability of postoperative results is high, in some cases, overcorrection and undercorrection can occur due to viscoelastic and biomechanics profile of the different keratoconic corneas.

The complications related to the ring itself are (1) halos and glare, (2) periannular deposits, and (3) neovascularization. Halos are reported by 10 % of patients and can be related to the pupil size. This symptom tends to fade or at least diminish over time. In very symptomatic cases, we usually prescribe pilocarpine or brimonidine tartarate at night, to constrict the pupil and alleviate the undesired reflexes. The periannular opacities are small white debris lying along the ring internal face. They do not tend to grow and do not harm visual performance, being only anti-esthetical when submitted to biomicroscopic examination. Neovascularization of the stromal tunnel is rare and usually occurs in atopic patients. We have used subconjunctival bevacizumab to treat this complication, with reasonable results, as reported by the literature [37–40].

Kwitiko et al. [8] reported FICR decentration in 3.9 % of cases, segment extrusion in 19.6 % and bacterial keratitis in 1.9 %. As the author mentioned in his paper, the surgeon's learning curve and different healing processes in keratoconic corneas can cause the majority of complications related to the surgical technique. Once the surgical procedure is mastered, the complications rate related to the surgery itself is very low. The surgical steps must be followed carefully (the stromal tunnel must be constructed with the adjustable diamond knife set at 80 % of local corneal thickness to reduce the chance of a shallow tunnel and subsequent ring extrusion) to avoid surgery-related complications.

As a general rule, it must be assumed that the thickest segment of a pair of segments cannot exceed half thickness of the cornea in its bed.

Based on our personal (unpublished) data, about 5 % of patients go to penetrating or lamellar keratoplasty due to progressive corneal scarring, despite proper FICR implantation. Some patients have a more aggressive form of ectasia, which can evolve even when treated early in the course of the disease.

2.13   Comments

Preliminary investigations have demonstrated that intracorneal rings are effective in the treatment of astigmatism and myopia with astigmatism [13], with preservation of BSCVA and stable results over time [14]. The objective of the addictive technology is to reinforce the cornea, decrease the corneal irregularity, and provide an improvement of the visual acuity in affected patients.

It is important to note an important reduction of keratometric values after the Ferrara ring implantation, with corneal regularization and return to its physiological values when the intervention is made early in the course of the disease. However, in a late intervention, with values of keratometry superior to 56D, it is also showed a reduction of the K, high keratometry values remain when compared to a normal corneal.

Our clinical findings are in agreement with other studies: Miranda et al. [41] obtained on their study a significant reduction in the mean central corneal curvature postoperatively. BSCVA and UCVA improved in 87.1 and 80.6 % of the eyes, respectively. Siganos et al. [16] showed an increase of the mean UCVA from 0.07 + 0.08 preoperatively to 0.20 + 0.13 and 0.30 + 0.21 after 1 and 6 months, respectively, and the mean BSCVA improved from 0.37 + 0.25 preoperatively to 0.50 + 0.43 and 0.60 + 0.17 after 1 and 6 months, respectively.

The Ferrara ring technique has the objective of reshaping the abnormal cornea, flattening the periphery, and decreasing the corneal astigmatism. With the objective to avoid, or at least postpone, the keratoplasty, the technique is within the options of visual rehabilitation of patients with keratoconus.

Observing the clinical outcomes of our patients, we could realize that the visual rehabilitation curve and refractive stabilization occurs on average, after three months of surgery. The visual rehabilitation process follows a certain pattern. In general, vision improvement is quick, and, on the day following surgery, the patients usually report subjective and objective improvement of the visual acuity. However, it usually reverts within the first weeks and at the end of the first month the patient reports that his/her vision was better immediately after surgery. The same fluctuation is detected in relation to refraction and keratometry. From the first month on, the vision starts to improve, and refractive and keratometric fluctuation decreases. From the third month on, it stabilizes. Then, it is possible to correct the residual ametropia, if necessary, by means of eyeglasses, rigid or soft contact lenses, or even implanting phakic intraocular lenses for high myopia correction.

We could notice that patients having central cones show a longer rehabilitation time, which means that the central flattening is slower, while patients with decentralized cones have faster rehabilitation. We believe this is due to the dislocation or the corneal apex toward its physiological position in front of the pupil. In some cases, we could observe that after the ring implantation there was an increase in myopia and in the keratometric readings, caused by this same phenomenon. As the 210-FICR study showed, the results in these types of cones, especially Nipple cones, are satisfactory.

The endothelial study showed that the Ferrara ring has minimal effect on the cornea endothelium. In our study we found a 1.4 % loss of endothelial cells per year. Considering that most of the studied patients were young, the rate of endothelial cell loss was slightly higher than in normal eyes (1.1 %). Moreover, there is no study in the current literature that shows the profile of the "normal" endothelial loss in keratoconus corneas, which could be higher than in normal corneas. The only report in the literature regarding the endothelium profile of keratoconus is non-prospective and studied only 12 eyes [32].

Symptoms like photophobia, visual discomfort, eye strain, and itching diminish or disappear after surgery.

Most of our patients are allergic; therefore, we recommend strongly that they should not rub their eyes, which could displace the segments and stimulate the disease progression. In addition, rubbing could theoretically change the regularity of the corneal surface leading to visual acuity loss. In some cases it will be necessary to use eye shields at night to prevent the patient from rubbing the eyes compulsively and unwarily.

The satisfaction level is high. We could observe that the fear of becoming blind in those patients, along with the fearsome possibility of a transplant in case of a continuously evolving condition, is very common. The possibility of postponing those eventualities generates great relief by the patients. Our cases show that, besides correcting the corneal deformity, the cone evolution is interrupted. Along with this interruption, we could also observe a decrease in corneal opacity and the other symptoms aforementioned.

The surgery is simple and well reproducible, although it is not an easy procedure. As in any other procedure, it must be well executed to attain a consistent result.

The incidence of complications is very low, around 3–5 %, compatible with the levels required for refractive procedures. It should be emphasized that the corneal ring implant is essentially an orthopedic technique designed to enable the correction of a structural deformity. As an advantage, it provides simultaneous refractive correction, although not well predictable, as with other refractive procedures.

The analysis of the results reveals that the visual rehabilitation without correction is satisfactory on initial stages of keratoconus (I and II), and it decreases in more advanced stages. "Nipple" type of keratoconus take longer to rehabilitate than those of the "sag" type. Conventional optical correction allows a high rate of visual correction—equal or greater than 20/60—and the resulting flattening enables the use of toric or spherical soft lenses, as well as refitting of rigid contact lenses, with an improvement in tolerance.

Whenever it was necessary to perform the keratoplasty, the ring not only helped the procedure but also provided a better centralization during trephination.

We could also notice that, after surgery, there was a decrease in the corneal sensitivity, resulting in greater comfort in contact lens fitting, which was not possible before the operation.

The incidence of complications is greater in more advanced stages, because the cornea is thinner, and the pressure generated inside the stroma after the ring implantation can cause the displacement of segments toward the incisions, eventually extruding the segments.

2.14   Conclusion

From the results obtained, we can state that this therapeutic approach has the following benefits:

1. Low morbidity, because it preserves the cornea structure and has a low rate of complications, allowing 95 % of the operated patients to quickly reintegrate themselves to their everyday activities.

2. Reversibility, because it enables the cornea to revert to the preoperative dimensions when the segments are removed.
3. Readjustability through segment replacement. In some cases, it was possible to correct hypercorrection removing just one of the segments.
4. Lack of rejection, the acrylic which the ring is made is inert and biocompatible.
5. Patients' high satisfaction rate.
6. As an orthopedic technique, it corrects corneal deformity and restores the physiologic curvature. After the surgery, it is possible to correct the residual ametropia with conventional optical correction or contact lenses.
7. Stabilization or delay of cone progression.
8. Lack of a minimum age for surgery, thus making it possible to reduce the wait lists for transplants in eye banks (30 % of the transplants in eye banks are attributed to keratoconus).
9. Possibility of association with other procedures like contact lens fitting and intraocular lenses.
10. No interference whatsoever with corneal transplant.

For all the reasons above, we believe the corneal intrastromal ring implant technique should be formally adopted as an extra option in treating corneal diseases which otherwise have had corneal transplant as a sole and ultimate solution.

2.15   Corneal Biomechanics

Cornea is a five-layered structure consisting of epithelium, Bowman's membrane, stroma, Descemet's membrane, and the endothelium. The epithelium and endothelium are not able to carry mechanical stress because of their cellular origin.

Bowman's and Descemet's membranes are about 10/im thick and contain collagen (type?). Bowman's membrane is composed of randomly oriented, loosely packed, small collagen fibrils surrounded by ground substance. The posterior surface merges with the superficial lamellae of the stroma to which it is firmly attached. In keratoconus breaks are frequently seen. But studies reported no significant difference in the elasticity of corneas with and without this layer both in corneal strips and inflation tests [42, 43]. In human inflation tests [44] the stress–strain curves did not change when Descemet's membrane was removed.

The stroma consists of about 300 lamellae (500 at limbus), each 15–25 μm thick and made up by collagen fibers embedded parallel to the surface in an amorphous matrix of glycosaminoglycans and proteoglycans. There is new evidence [45] that the lamellae split in anteroposterior direction as well as horizontally into branches and are interlaced by crossing the fissures between the branches. The anterior lamellae are bundle shaped, thinner, and closely packed. The cross angles varied between 1 and 90° with the exception of the limbal region close to the Descemet's membrane (ligamentum circulare corneae) where the angles are lower than 30°. These findings were deduced biomechanically by measuring the cohesive strength of the cornea [46] and do not contradict the evidence that the surface of the cornea can slide relative to one another but limited to these interlamellar ties.

The less packed posterior stroma could give a certain relaxation under no stress or less stiffness under physiological stress. This produces a j-shape nonlinear stress–strain behavior but heterogeneous where the anterior stroma is stiffer than the posterior.

In keratoconus, it is believed that a loss of cohesion between collagen fibrils and the matrix produces a slippage of the lamellae that produces the ectasia and thinning. This loss of cohesion can be produced biochemically as it is reported (refs). The basis of this biomechanical hypothesis is the change of preferential orientation in keratoconus and a redistribution of mass (not a loss, except in advanced keratoconus).

2.16   Corneal Modelling

A number of studies have been undertaken in an attempt to characterize the mechanical properties of the cornea. The corneal biomechanics has been described by in vitro simple tension [42, 47–50], inflation [43, 44, 51–53], and compression tests [54]. The biomechanical response of the cornea in surgical procedures has been described by measuring local deformations [55–57]. Others have used finite element models with different assumptions regarding corneal geometry and material properties. Some have assumed that the cornea is a homogeneous linear elastic [58–60], nonlinear elastic [52, 57, 61, 62] solid, and a nonhomogeneous membrane [63].

Attempts to verify these models have been done with inflations tests [52] in hydrated corneas and with local deformations [57] in normo-hydrated corneas. The relationship between corneal strain and intraocular pressure was found to be nonlinear, showing a typical stress-stiffening behavior. A material model by Woo et al. [51] has been used to account that nonlinearity [52, 57, 62].

2.17   Anisotropy

The anisotropy of the cornea is evidenced by its microstructure as a reinforced composite with collagen fibers immersed in a jellylike matrix of mucopolysaccharides. Meek et al. map the collagen orientation in normal and keratoconus corneas [64]. They found that a preferred orientation in the inf–sup and nasal–temporal directions in the central posterior stroma gradually changed from 2 mm to a circumferential orientation at the limbus. In chickens this anisotropy is maximum and declines progressively with developing age [65].

There have been attempts to account the anisotropy of the cornea in a model, with transverse isotropy but since the cornea is also nearly incompressible [54] violates the restrictions on the elastic constants. Pinsky et al. modeled the anisotropy produced by the relaxing incisions in a thick membrane model. But local bending effects near the incision were found to be an important factor [57]. Further extensions in a 3D model have been presented where a transverse isotropic model of the fibrils and a rotational averaging at the corneal plane give an adequate treatment of the anisotropy of the stroma [1].

2.18 Viscoelasticity

The hydration has a profound effect on the extensibility of the stroma [57]. But these effects are minimal in the anterior stroma [66] even under extreme conditions of hydration. The viscoelastic effects of the cornea have been measured in inflations tests [67], in corneal strips [42], and in cylindrical corneal samples [68]. In vivo properties were measured by Buzard et al. after refractive procedures [69]. A complete model of the cornea should take into account the poroelasticity, viscoelasticity, and anisotropicity of the cornea.

2.19 Nonlinearity

Hyperelastic models are proper for material and geometric nonlinearities. Geometric nonlinearities appear in inflation tests as well as in refractive procedures like those involving the insertion of intrastromal rings. They are also suitable for further extension to anisotropy and viscoelasticity. There were attempts to use rubber-based hyperelastic models, like Mooney–Rivlin [52, 70] and Ogden [52], but they did not reproduce the high nonlinearity of the cornea.

Several authors proposed to use exponential material models to represent the nonlinear elastic behavior of biological tissues. For instance, Fung proposed the following strain energy:

$$W = \frac{\mu_0}{2\gamma}\left[e^{\gamma(I_1-3)} - 1\right] \tag{5.1}$$

where μ_0 (shear modulus), γ are positive material constants [71, 72], and I_1 is a measure of the strain (first invariant). Also, Woo et al. [51] used an exponential model, in small strains, to analyze the corneal stroma, sclera, and optic nerve:

$$\sigma_{\text{eff}} = \alpha\left(e^{\beta\varepsilon_{\text{eff}}} - 1\right) \tag{5.2}$$

where σ_{eff} and ε_{eff} are effective stress and strain, respectively, and α and β are material constants. Bryant et al. used a similar model and characterized its parameters in an inflation test after failing with a rubber-based Mooney–Rivlin and Ogden hyperelastic models. This model accounts the material nonlinearity but is not suitable for further developments of viscoelasticity, as it was proposed in [4].

An hyperelastic exponential model was proposed, with an integral of the exponential term, in order to have a simpler form in the stress and elasticity matrix, after differentiation. A second logarithmic term was added with the second invariant of the deformation tensor C (similar to the Hart–Smith model) and a third logarithmic term with the third invariant of the deformation tensor C to account the nearly incompressibility [73].

The strain energy function W results in

$$W(I_1, I_2, I_3) = c_1 \int e^{c_3(I_1 - 3)} dI_1 + c_2 \ln \frac{I_2}{3} + 2c_4(I_3 - 1) + c_5(\ln I_3)^2 \qquad (5.3)$$

with material constants c_1, c_2, c_3, c_4 and c_5. Details of this model are described elsewhere [74]. This model is isotropic and is the base where the anisotropic model is developed.

2.20 Anisotropic Model

In order to account the anisotropic properties of the stroma, a transverse- isotropic model with rotational averaging was proposed by Pinsky and Guarnieri [1]. A model for a typical lamella is created and then a cornea model by averaging the lamella model through the stroma. The strain energy density is assumed to be additively decomposed into three parts:

1. The part W_T describes the isotropic ground substance.
2. The part W_L describes the collagen fibrils with orientation **a**.
3. The part W_C describes the fibril–fibril cross-linking and fibril–ground substance interaction.

$$W = W_T + W_L + W_C \qquad (5.4)$$

where

$$W_L = \frac{1}{4} \beta \left[\int e^{\gamma(I_4 - 1)} dI_4 - 1 \right] \qquad (5.5)$$

and W_T is described by an isotropic hyperelastic model (like Mooney–Rivlin) and W_C is described by a linear form which satisfies energy restrictions.

Assuming random orientation of the lamellae in the corneal plane, a rotational averaging of the energy density function of the form is introduced (Fig. 5.6)

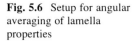

Fig. 5.6 Setup for angular averaging of lamella properties

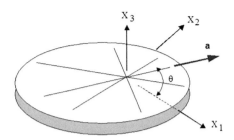

$$W' = \frac{1}{\pi}\int_0^\pi \Phi(x,\theta)W(a)d\theta \qquad (5.6)$$

where each vector a provides the dependence on θ (in fact $\theta = \arctan(\alpha_2 = \alpha_1)$), and $\Phi(\theta)$ is a weighting function of θ which can be used to describe nonuniform angular distribution of lamellae in different regions of the cornea (e.g., preferential orientation at the limbus) (see [75]).

3 Modeling Intacs

The cornea was idealized as an astigmatic cornea with two principal radii of curvature. Proper limbal conditions were set where the limbus can move freely in the thickness direction. Details of the geometry and boundary conditions can be obtained at [74].

A quarter of the cornea was modeled using hexahedral finite elements with 27 nodes. The mesh of elements is structured, and proper refining was used on the channel to obtain good convergence without compromising computational analysis time. Since the geometry is a quarter (see Fig. 5.7), there is symmetry at the x and y planes. The segment is cut half in the y plane and is free to move in this plane but not in the y direction. This symmetry is enough for astigmatic cases, and the incision effect is not taken into account.

The intraocular pressure was set to 16 mmHg. The constitutive law used was described above. Standard contact boundary conditions were applied between the segment and the tissue of the channel.

The results of the simulation are shown in Fig. 5.7. In Fig. 5.8a, the magnitude of displacement is shown (maximum red). The change of curvature was −0.9/+0.8 D in the y plane (segment) and the x plane, respectively. In Fig. 5.8b, a thicker segment (0.35 mm) was used with 120° of arc. The change of refraction was −8.1/+0.9.

Fig. 5.7 A 3D quarter
model of the interaction
between a segment implant
and the cornea

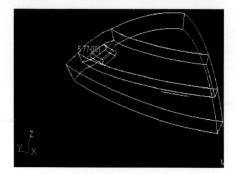

4 Modeling Ferrara Rings for Astigmatism

A Ferrara ring segment was modeled and compared with an Intacs for a segment thickness of 0.20 mm and 90° of arc. The magnitude of displacement plot for the Ferrara ring segment is shown in Fig. 5.9. Note the displacement of the interior edge to the apex and the rotation through the segment axis clockwise.

The change of refraction for both segments (Intacs and Ferrara) was −2.7/+0.1 D and −3.4/+0.2 D, respectively. Clearly, the Ferrara ring produced a higher correction.

The Ferrara ring segments are inserted in a smaller optical zone of 6 mm (instead of 8.1 mm) and narrower channel width between 0.65 and 1 mm. The change of refraction for this optical zone was −12/0.28 D for a channel width of 0.9 mm and −16/0.50 for 0.8 mm.

In Figs. 5.10 and 5.11, the simulation of a Ferrara ring segment of 0.30 mm and 160° of arc with an optical zone of 0.6 mm is shown.

The change of refraction was extremely higher (−15.5/0.25 D) with a channel width of 1.0 mm.

4.1 Heterogeneity of the Cornea

Considering the mechanical behavior caused by the differential organization of the lamella, the model is based where the material is more rigid anteriorly (300 MPa) and less rigid posteriorly (30 MPa). This heterogeneity of the material allowed obtaining refractive results closer to clinical findings for normal corneas. A 0.20 mm ring segment with 120° of arc was simulated with these heterogeneous material parameters. Figs. 5.11 and 5.12 show the magnitude of displacements, and the refractive change obtained was −2.3/0.15 D.

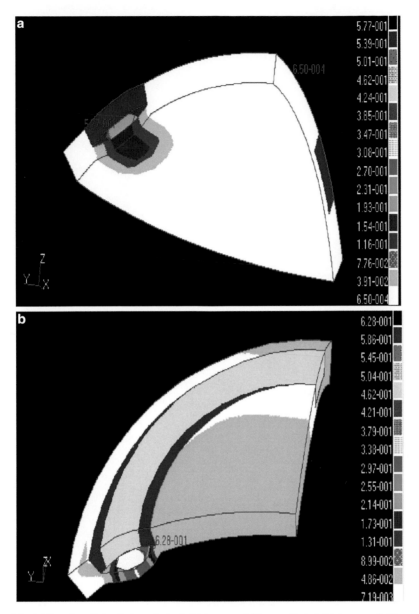

Fig. 5.8 (**a**) Results of simulation. Apical thickness = 0.52 mm; limbal thickness = 0.65 mm; K vertical = 48.3D;   K   horizontal = 46.3D;   diameter   (vertical) = 10.5   mm;   diameter horizontal = 11.5 mm; segment thickness = 0.20 mm; segment arc = 30°; optical zone = 8.1 mm; channel width = 1.5 mm (**b**) a thicker segment (0.35 mm) was used with 120 of arc

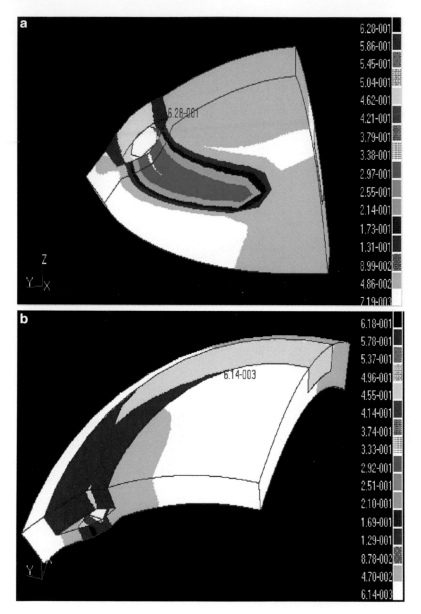

Fig. 5.9 (a) An Intacs ring segment (b) A Ferrara ring segment both with thickness of 0.20 mm and 90 of arc

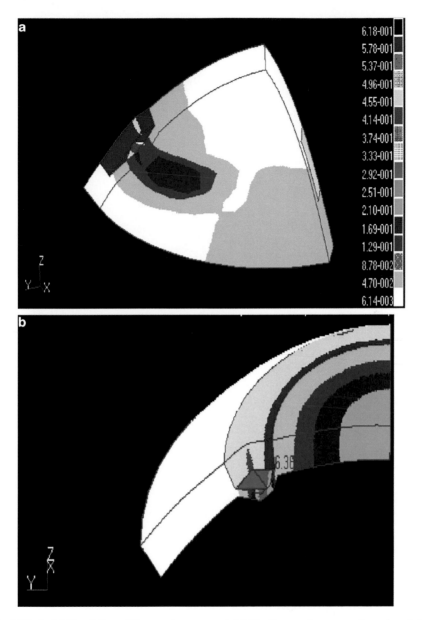

Fig. 5.10 (**a**, **b**) Simulation of Ferrara ring segment. (a) The Ferrara ring segments are inserted in an optical zone of 8.1 mm (b) optical zone of 6 mm and narrower channel width (below 1 mm)

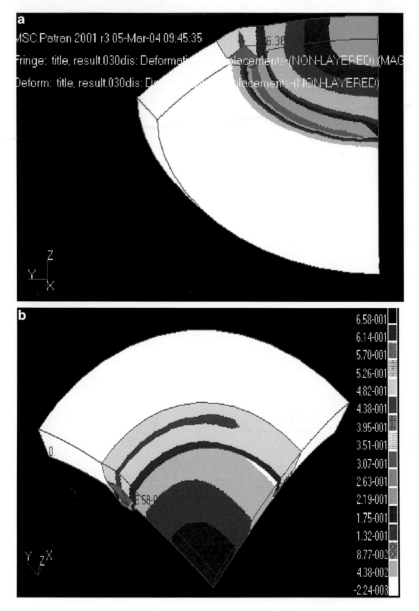

Fig. 5.11 (**a, b**) Simulation of a Ferrara ring segment of 0.30 mm and 160 of arc with an optical zone of 0.6 mm

Fig. 5.12 Magnitude of displacement and refractive change obtained where the material is more rigid anteriorly (300 MPa) and less rigid posteriorly (30 MPa)

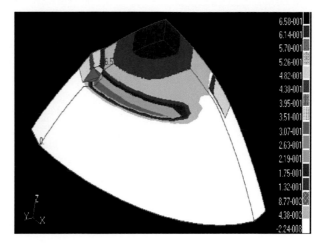

5   Modeling Ferrara Rings for Keratoconus

Pentacam corneal data as pachymetric, elevation, and topography maps were obtained from keratoconus patients (Fig. 5.13). The corneal geometry was reconstructed based on keratometric and pachymetric data. The cone was simulated by weakening the corneal material centered at the cone apex and extended to a cone radius based on elevation map (Fig. 5.14). The surgery with Ferrara asymmetric rings was simulated with a finite element model as described in previous analysis. The elevation map of the simulation is shown in Fig. 5.15. By comparing this map with the elevation map postsurgery there is a clear agreement between both maps. The cone is reduced in the simulation by −45 µm. An increase in the elevation is produced peripherally at the ends of both rings (at 115 meridian) of +31 µm. In the real surgery an elevation at the cone of +105 µm is reduced to +35 um (total −75 µm), and a depression of −161 at 115 meridian is elevated to −56 µm (total +105 µm). The model shows the tendency but is a little stiff, mainly caused by still unknown parameters like healing and elasticity of tissue.

> **Conclusions**
>
> It was described the biomechanics of the cornea and the modeling and simulation with intracorneal segments, Intacs and Ferrara.
>
> The corneal model was described considering new findings in the ultra-structure of the stroma like the interlamellar ties and interweaving of the lamella. This does not contradict the relative sliding that is found between each pair of adjacent lamella that is given by the model as a low value of shear stiffness. A viscohyperelastic model is adapted to this heterogeneity of the material causing different properties for the anterior and posterior stroma (Figs. 5.13, 5.14, 5.15, and 5.16).

(continued)

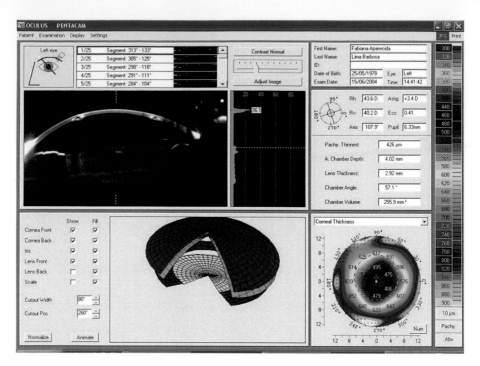

Fig. 5.13 Pentacam corneal data (pachymetric, elevation, and topography maps)obtained from a keratoconus patient

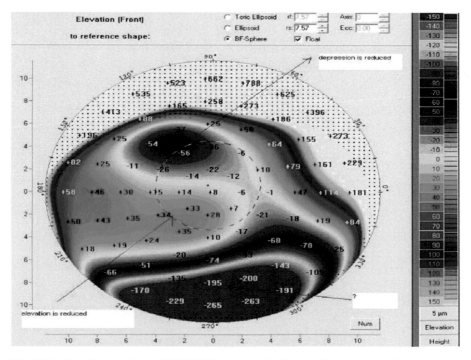

Fig. 5.14 Elevation map from PENTACAM showing the highest depression and elevation

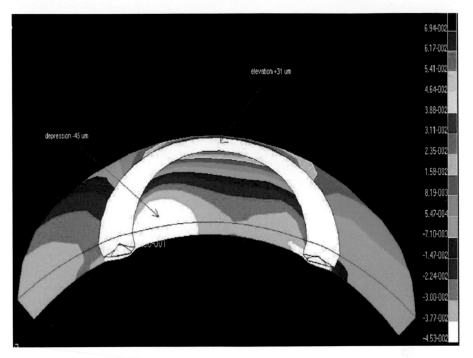

Fig. 5.15 The surgery with Ferrara asymmetric rings was simulated with a finite element model. Elevation is shown with colored scale. See highest depression and elevation obtained by simulation and compared with PENTACAM postop (Fig 5.16)

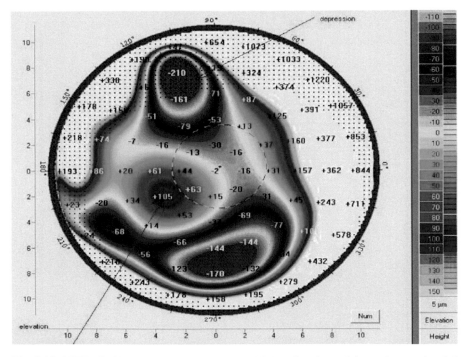

Fig. 5.16 PENTACAM elevation map postsurgery. Highest elevation and depression are signaled

(continued)

Intacs segments are modeled and compared with Ferrara segments with the optical zone and channel width used in Intacs. For an 8.1 mm optical zone and a channel width of 1.5 mm, the refractive power of the Ferrara segments were higher.

The channel width in Ferrara rings was an important parameter given the nonplanar contact between the base of the segment and the inferior side of the channel. Variations of 0.2 mm in the channel width gave more than 2 diopters of difference.

The elasticity of the cornea is also a sensible parameter of the refractive outcome. An initial 9 MPa value obtained from previous work [74] was used. But the refractive change obtained was too high comparing clinical results with Intacs and Ferrara rings. The heterogeneity of the cornea was taken into account in the model, and a more rigid anterior stroma and a less rigid posterior stroma gave results closer to clinical findings.

More studies should be done considering the compressive properties of the cornea.

A keratoconic cornea was simulated by using Pentacam geometrical data and simulating the cone by weakening the corneal material in the zone under the cone. A similar behavior was obtained with the postelevation maps (a reduction of the height of the cone and an elevation at the ends of the rings). Unknown elastic and healing parameters would improve these preliminary results. Further studies are being performed in order to increase the number of cases simulated and to obtain the elastic and healing parameters from in vivo patients.

The introduced model is an interesting tool for new designs of the surgery and rings. The Ferrara nomogram used today differentiate different types of keratoconus (see Fig. 5.4), and this model would be capable to improve this nomogram by precise selection of location, length of arc, and thickness of rings based on pachymetry, topography, and elevation maps of each patient and not using nomograms based on empirical modifications and regression analysis.

Acknowledgments This work was partly funded by Ferrara Rings, Inc. (Belo Horizonte, Brazil). I would like to thank Dr. Paulo Ferrara for his support and collaboration of this work.

References

1. F.A. Guarnieri, P.M. Pinsky, J. Shimmick, Computational investigation of the biomechanical response of the cornea to lamellar procedures. Invest. Ophthalmol. Vis. Sci. **42**, S603 (2001)
2. T.A. Silvestrini, M.L. Mathis, B.E. Loomas, T.E. Burris, A geometric model to predict the change in corneal curvature from the intrastromal corneal ring (ICR). Invest. Ophthalmol. Vis. Sci. **35**(suppl), 2023 (1994)

3. P.M. Pinsky, D.V. Datye, T.A. Silvestrini, Numerical simulation of topographical alterations in the cornea after ICR (intrastromal corneal ring) placement. Invest. Ophthalmol. Vis. Sci. **36** (suppl), S309 (1995)
4. F.A. Guarnieri, A. Cardona, 3d viscoelastic nonlinear incompressible finite element in large strain of the cornea. application in refractive surgery, in *Articles in CD-ROM Fourth World Congress of Computational Mechanics* (1998)
5. J. Colin, S. Velou, Implantation of intacs and a refractive intraocular lens to correct keratoconus. J. Cataract Refract. Surg. **29**(4), 832–834 (2003)
6. P.A. Asbell, Ó.m.Ó. Ugakhan, Long-term follow-up of intacs from a single center. J. Cataract Refract. Surg. **27**(9), 1456–1468 (2001)
7. J. Colin, B. Cochener, G. Savary et al., Correcting keratoconus with intra-corneal rings. J. Cataract Refract. Surg. **26**, 1117–1122 (2000)
8. D. Siganos, P. Ferrara, K. Chatzinikolas et al., Ferrara intrastromal corneal rings for the correction of keratoconus. J. Cataract Refract. Surg. **28**, 1947–1951 (2002)
9. J. Colin, B. Cochener, G. Savary et al., Intacs inserts for treating keratoconus; one-year results. Ophthalmology **108**, 1409–1414 (2001)
10. C.S. Siganos, G.D. Kymionis, N. Kartakis et al., Management of keratoconus with Intacs. Am. J. Ophthalmol. **135**, 64–70 (2003)
11. K.K. Assil, A.M. Barrett, B.D. Fouraker, D.J. Schanzlin, One-year results of the intrastromal corneal ring in nonfunctional human eyes; the Intrastromal Corneal Ring Study Group. Arch. Ophthalmol. **113**, 159–167 (1995)
12. C.S. Siganos, G.D. Kymionis, N. Astyrakakis et al., Management of corneal ectasia after laser in situ keratomileusis with INTACS. J. Refract. Surg. **18**, 43–46 (2002)
13. F.B.D. Silva, E.A.F. Alves, P.F.A. Cunha, Utilizagao do Anel de Ferrara na estabilizagdo e corregao da ectasia corneana pós PRK. Arq. Bras. Oftalmol. **63**, 215–218 (2000)
14. J. Ruckhofer, J. Stoiber, M.D. Twa et al., Correction of astigmatism with short arc-length intrastromal corneal ring segments: preliminary results. Ophthalmology **110**, 516–524 (2003)
15. W. Nose, R.A. Neves, T.E. Burris et al., Intrastromal corneal ring: 12-month sighted myopic eyes. J. Refract. Surg. **12**, 20–28 (1996)
16. D.J. Schanzlin, P.A. Asbell, T.E. Burris, D.S. Durrie, The intrastromal ring segments; phase II results for the correction of myopia. Ophthalmology **104**, 1067–1078 (1997)
17. D.K. Holmes-Higgin, T.E. Burris, J.A: Lapidus, M.R. Greenlick, Risk factors for self-reported visual symptoms with Intacs inserts for myopia. Ophthalmology **109**, 46–56 (2002)
18. P.A. Asbell, O. Ucakhan, R.L. Abbott et al., Intrastromal corneal ring segments: reversibility of refractive effect. J. Refract. Surg. **17**, 25–31 (2001)
19. J.I. Barraquer, Modification of refraction by means of intracorneal inclusions. Int. Ophthalmol. Clin. **6**(1), 53–78 (1966)
20. J.L. Barraquer, *Cirugia Refractiva de La Cornea* (Instituto Barraquer de America, Bogota, Tomo I, 1989)
21. J.I. Barraquer, Modification of refraction by means of intracorneal inclusion. Int. Ophthamol. Clin. **6**, 53 (1966)
22. P. Ferrara, L. Torquetti, Clinical outcomes after implantation of a new intrastromal ring with a 210-degree of arch. J. Cataract Refract. Surg. **35**, 1604–1608 (2009)
23. L. Torquetti, P. Ferrara, Long term follow-up of intrastromal corneal ring segments in keratoconus. J. Cataract Refract. Surg. **35**, 1768–1773 (2009)
24. P. Ferrara, L. Torquetti, Ferrara Ring, *An Overview.* Cataract and Refractive Surgery Today Ü Europe (2009)
25. A. Ertan, G. Kamburoglu, Ü. Akgun, Comparison of outcomes of 2 channel sizes for intrastromal ring segment implantation with a femtosecond laser in eyes with keratoconus. J. Cataract Refract. Surg. **33**, 648–653 (2007)
26. A. Ertan, G. Kamburoglu, M. Bahadir, Intacs insertion with the femtosecond laser for the management of keratoconus: one-year results. J. Cataract Refract. Surg. **32**, 2039–2042 (2006)
27. Y.S. Rabinowitz, X. Li, T.S. Ignacio, E. Maguen, Intacs inserts using the femtosecond laser compared to the mechanical spreader in the treatment of keratoconus. J. Refract. Surg. **22**, 764–771 (2006)

28. M.H. Shabayek, J.L. Alió, Intrastromal corneal ring segment implantation by femtosecond laser for keratoconus correction. Ophthalmology 114, 1643–1652 (2007)
29. P.M. Pinsky, D. van der Heide, D. Chernyak, Computational modeling of mechanical anisot-317 ropy in the cornea and sclera. J. Cataract Refract. Surg. 31(1), 136–145 (2005)
30. L. Torquetti, P. Ferrara, Intrastromal corneal ring segments implantation in post-refractive surgery ectasia. J. Cataract Refract. Surg. 36, 986–990 (2010)
31. P. Ferrara, L. Torquetti, Corneal endothelial profile after Ferrara ring implantation. J. Emmetropia 1, 29–32 (2010)
32. W.M. Bourne, L.R. Nelson, D.O. Hodge, Continued endothelial cell loss ten years after implantation. Ophthalmology 101, 1014–1023 (1994)
33. R.A. Laing, M.M. Sandstrom, A.R. Berrospi, H.M. Leibowitz, The human corneal endothelium in keratoconus: a specular microscopic study. Arch. Ophthalmol. 97, 1867–1869 (1979)
34. Langenbucher A, Nguyen NX, and Seitz B. *Predictive donor factors for chronic endothelial cell loss after nonmechanical penetrating keratoplasty in a regression model.* GraefeSs Arch Clin Exp Ophtalmol, 2003.
35. Azar RG, Holdbrook MJ, Lemp M, and Edelhauser HF; KeraVision Stduy Group. *Two-year corneal endothelial cell assessment following INTACS implantation.* J Refract Surg, 2001.
36. G Wollensak, Spoerl E, Wilsch M, and Seiler T. *Endothelial cell damage after riboflavin-ultraviolet-A treatment in the rabbit.* J Cataract Refract Surg 2003;29:1786–1790.
37. Dastjerdi MH, Al-Arfaj KM, Nallasamy N, Hamrah P, and Jurkunas UV. *Pineda R 2nd.* Pavan-Langston D, Dana R, Topical bevacizumab in the treatment of corneal neovascularization, 2009.
38. Mackenzie SE, Tucker WR, and Poole TR. *Bevacizumab (avastin) for corneal neovascularization-corneal light shield soaked application.* Cornea, 2009.
39. Chen WL, Lin CT, Lin NT, Tu IH, Li JW, Chow LP, Liu KR, and Hu FR. *Subconjunctival injection of bevacizumab (avastin) on corneal neovascular- ization in different rabbit models of corneal angiogenesis.* Invest Ophthalmol Vis Sci, 2009.
40. Doctor PP, Bhat PV, and Foster CS. *Subconjunctival bevacizumab for corneal neovascularization.* Cornea, 2008.
41. Miranda D, Sartori M, Francesconi C, Allemann N, Ferrara P, and Campos M. *Ferrara intrastromal corneal ring segments for severe keratoconus.* J Refract Surg, 2003.
42. T. Seiler, M. Matallana, S. Sendler, T. Bende, Does bowman's layer determine the biomechanical properties of the cornea? Refract. Corneal Surg. 8(2), 139–142 (1992)
43. J. 0. Hjortdal and N. Ehlers. Extensibility of the normo-hydrated human cornea. Acta Ophthalmol. Scand., 73(1):12–17, 1995.
44. B. Jue, D. Maurice, The mechanical properties of the rabbit and human cornea. J Biomechanics 19(10), 847–854 (1986)
45. R. Aufreiter, R. Mallinger, W. Radner, M. Zehetmayer, Interlacing and cross-angle distribution of collagen lamellae in the human cornea. Cornea 17(5), 537–543 (1998)
46. M.K. Smolek, Interlamellar cohesive strength in the vertical meridian of human eye bank corneas. Invest. Ophthalmol. Vis. Sci. 34(10), 2962–2969 (1993)
47. J. Gloster, E. S. Perkins, and M-L Pommier. Extensibility of strips of sclera and cornea. *British. J. Ophthal.*, 41:103–110, 1957.
48. A. Arciniegas and L. E. Amaya. *Asociación de la queratotomía radial y la circular para la corrección de ametropias. Enfoque biomecánico,* chapter XXII. Soc. Am. de Oftalmología, Bogotá, 1981.
49. I.S. Nash, P.R. Greene, C.S. Foster, Comparison of mechanical properties of keratoconus and normal corneas. Exp. Eye Res. 35, 413–423 (1982)
50. D.A. Hoeltzel, P. Altman, K.A. Buzard, K. Choe, Strip extensiometry for comparison of the mechanical response of bovine, rabbit and human corneas. J Biomech Engng 114(2), 202–215 (1992)
51. S.L.-Y. Woo, A.S. Kobayashi, W.A. Schlegel, C. Lawrence, Nonlinear material properties of intact cornea and sclera. Exp. Eye Res. 14, 29–39 (1972)

52. M.R. Bryant, P.J. McDonnell, Constitutive laws for biomechanical modeling of refractive surgery. J Biomech Engng **118**, 473–481 (1996)
53. A. Nevyas-Wallace. Pattern recognition in subclinical and clinical kerato- conus using elevation-based topography. In *Abstracts in Pre-AAO. ISRS*, page 98, 1996.
54. J.L. Battaglioli, R.D. Kamm, Measurements of the compressive prop- erties of scleral tissue. Invest. Ophthalmol. Vis. Sci. **114**(2), 202–215 (1992)
55. K.A. Buzard, J.F. Ronk, M.H. Friedlander, D.J. Tepper, D.A. Hoeltzel, K. Choe, Quantitative measurement of wound spreading in radial keratotomy. Refract. Corneal Surg. **8**(3), 217–223 (1992)
56. J. 0. Hjortdal and N. Ehlers. Acute tissue deformation of the human cornea after radial keratotomy. J. Refract. Surg., 12(3):391–400, 1996.
57. W.M. Petroll, P. Roy, C.J. Chuong, B. Hall, H.D. Cavanagh, J.V. Jester, Measurement of surgically induced corneal deformations us- ing three-dimensional confocal microscopy. Cornea **15**(2), 154–164 (1996)
58. R.P. Vito, P.H. Carnell, Finite element method based mechanical models of the cornea for pressure and indenter loading. Refract. Corneal Surg. **8**(2), 146–151 (1992)
59. S.C. Velinsky, M.R. Bryant, On the computer-aided and optimal design of keratorefractive surgery. Refract. Corneal Surg. **8**(2), 173–182 (1992)
60. F. A. Guarnieri. Modelo biomecánico del ojo para diseño asistido por computadora de la cirugía refractiva. Proyecto de grado de bioingeniería, Facultad de Ingeniería, UNER, Oro Verde, Entre Ríos, Argentina, 1993.
61. K. D. Hanna, F. E. Jouve, and G. O. Waring(III). Computer simulation of arcuate keratotomy for astigmatism. *Refract. Corneal Surg.,* 8(2):152–163, 1992.
62. W. O. Wray, E. D. Best, and L. Y. Cheng. A mechanical model for radial keratotomy: Toward a predictive capability. J. *Biomech. Engng.,* 116(1), 1994.
63. P.M. Pinsky, D.V. Datye, Numerical modeling of radial, astigmatic and hexagonal keratotomy. Refract. Corneal Surg. **8**(2), 164–172 (1992)
64. K.M. Meek, S.J. Tuft, Y. Huang, P.S. Gill, S. Hayes, R.H. Newton, A.J. Bron, Changes in collagen orientation and distribution in keratoconus corneas. Invest. Ophthalmol. Vis. Sci. **46**, 1948–1956 (2005)
65. A.J. Quantock, C. Boote, V. Siegler, K.M. Meek, Collagen organization in the secondary chick cornea during development. Invest. Ophthalmol. Vis. Sci. **44**, 130–136 (2003)
66. L.J. Müller, E. Pels, G.F.J.M. Vrensen, The specific architecture of the anterior stroma accounts for maintenance of corneal curvature. Br. J. Ophthalmol. **85**, 437–443 (2001)
67. A.S. Kobayashi, L.G. Staberg, W.A. Schlegel, Viscoelastic properties of human cornea. Exp. Mech. **13**(12), 497–503 (1973)
68. M.K. Smolek, Holographic interferometry of intact and radially incised human eye-bank corneas. J. Cataract Refract. Surg. **20**, 277–286 (1994)
69. K.A. Buzard, B.R. Fundingsland, Assessment of corneal wound healing by interactive topog- raphy. J. Refract. Surg. **14**, 53–60 (1998)
70. K.D. Hanna, F.E. Jouve, G.O. Waring III, Preliminary computer simulation of the effects of radial keratotomy. Arch. Ophthalmol. **107**, 911–918 (1989)
71. M.F. Beatty, Topics in finite elasticity: hyperelasticity of rubber, elastomers, and biological tissues- with examples. Appl. Mech. Rev. **40**, 1699–1734 (1987)
72. Y.C. Fung, *Biomechanics. Mechanical Properties of Living Tissues*, 2nd edn. (Springer, New York, 1993)
73. A.D. Drozdov, *Finite Elasticity and Viscoelasticity. A Course in the Nonlinear Mechanics of Solids* (World Scientific, Singapore, 1996)
74. F. A. Guarnieri. *Modelo Biomecánico del Ojo para Diseño Asistido por Computadora de la Cirugía Refractiva. PhD* dissertation, FICH-INTEC, Universidad Nacional del Litoral, Santa Fe, Argentina, 1999.
75. P.M. Pinsky, D. van der Heide, D. Chernyak, Computational modeling of mechanical anisot- 317 ropy in the cornea and sclera. J. Cataract Refract. Surg. **31**(1), 136–145 (2005)

Chapter 6
Biomechanical Instrumentation in Refractive Surgery

Fabio A. Guarnieri and Andrés Guzmán

1 Intraocular Pressure (IOP) and Its Measurement: Tonometry

Ophthalmology is a branch of medicine science that studies the eye as a whole (anatomy, physiology, strength, health). One issue in ophthalmology is the accurate measurement of the intraocular pressure (IOP) due to its influence on several ophthalmology diseases (e.g., glaucoma).

The hypotheses that relate ocular diseases with IOP evoke several researchers as Goldmann to perform analytical and experimental studies focused to determine the IOP levels where it can be harmful for the visual field [1]. It is considered that a normal IOP ranges between 10 and 21 mmHg; the average value is 16 ± 2 mmHg [2]. Persistent values above 21 mmHg are considered as ocular hypertension.

The ocular hypertension is considered as one of the main factors conducing to damage in the ocular structures, glaucoma-damage on the retina and optical nerve head, loss of visual field due to neuronal death, and finally, irreversible blindness.

As stated before, the glaucoma is a silent and irreversible illness where the IOP produces damage to the optical nerve fibers. The symptoms are, at the beginning, lateral visual field loss, and central visual field loss in advanced stages. Glaucoma is characterized by IOP increase, hardening of the eye globe, and atrophy of optic papilla. The blindness is the worst consequence. There is a genetic link for this kind of illness.

F.A. Guarnieri, Ph.D. (✉)
Department of Bioengineering, Centro de Investigación de Métodos
Computacionales (CIMEC), Predio CONICET-Santa Fe, Colectora Ruta Nac 168,
Km 472, Paraje El Pozo, 3000 Santa Fe, Argentina
e-mail: aguarni@santafe-conicet.gov.ar

A. Guzmán, Ph.D.
Universidad del Norte, Barranquilla, Atlantico, Colombia

If a patient exam reports an IOP of above 25–30 mmHg, he or she will be on visual field loss risk if this pressure is sustained for long periods. Nevertheless, high IOPs could cause blindness in days or even hours. As IOP increases, the optic nerve axons are compressed in the spot where they leave the ocular globe at the optic disc. This compressive load causes an alteration on nutrition mechanisms of the optic nerve fibers and this will lead to death of these cells. In most cases, elevated IOPs generate a high resistance on the exit of effluent through the trabecular spaces of the Schlemm's canal in the iridocorneal angle.

The glaucoma progression is controlled by application of medicated eye drops that diffuse inside the eye globe. The eye drops effects could be the reduction of secretion of the aqueous humor or an increase of its absorption. If the medicated therapy is not effective as desired, it is necessary to apply surgical techniques that open spaces inside the trabecular meshwork facilitating the drainage from inside the eye to the subconjunctival space, outside the eye globe, reducing the IOP.

The most common procedure to measure pressure quantities is the manometry. A manometer is an instrument that visually indicates the pressure state of a fluid (gas or liquid). A direct manometry could be performed through a glass tube with a "U" shape filled with distilled water. In this procedure, the tube will have in a branch, a higher column of water due to pressure difference (exceeding the atmospheric pressure) if the medium where the pressure is measured has a positive pressure (no vacuum). Despite being a good device to measure pressure quantities with exactitude it lacks a wide range of measurements and it has a sensibility to the environment (the atmospheric pressure depends on the altitude above sea level in m.a.s.l.).

The IOP is the pressure within the ocular globe; this pressure assures the tone of the globe. The internal liquid (aqueous or vitreous humor) has the function to transport nutrients inside the ocular tissues and regulate cellular processes, in addition to its structural function. Also, the IOP could be defined as the result of the dynamic balance between the formation and evacuation of aqueous humor; this balance is possible under normal conditions [3].

Tonometry is each indirect procedure for measure the fluid pressure inside the eye (IOP). This procedure was initiated since nineteenth century. The theory behind the tonometry is subjected to a wide number of restrictions due to the way the mathematical and physical theories were applied and how the experiments were performed. These restrictions have as a consequence a low range of application; this technique is only appropriate for adult healthy eyes. Nevertheless, this technique is the only one for a fast and practical determination of the IOP.

From the engineering point of view, as a support field to the understanding of the mechanical behavior of the cornea, it is necessary to establish the geometrical parameters for the cornea, additional to its physical and functional characteristics. The geometrical parameters that influence the ocular globe behavior are correlated with population characteristics as race, age, and refractive antecedents.

It is important to remind the reader that mechanical and functional parameters for the cornea are functions of the patient's age. That is why some researchers have performed studies regarding this variation [4–11] and also have developed calibration equations from statistical analysis [12–18].

Fig. 6.1 Loading condition for tonometry

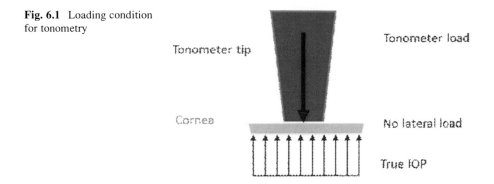

Functional parameters for the cornea include boundary conditions for the eye: IOP (load) and scleral limbus (restraints). In tonometry, we include another loading condition: pressure from the tonometer (Fig. 6.1).

Several years ago, the tonometry has been reviewed due to some difficulties detected on its fundamentals: design of the equipment, theory behind its development, and suppositions in the measure [12, 15, 18–28]. The Goldmann tonometry as a standard was calibrated with healthy adult eyes [3, 29]; that's why now, it is not recommended for application in children [1].

1.1 Tonometry Exam: Procedure

All contact tonometers work according to the same basis: Imbert's Law [29, 30]. Imbert's Law establishes that if we have a circular tissue with an insignificant thickness (elastic membrane behavior) loaded in its internal face (the sphere is filled with fluid), it is possible to measure the internal pressure, applying a variable force against the external face in a known area until equilibrium is reached. In this sense, the tonometer mechanism intends to flatten a corneal region producing a known circular area.

This law (or theory?) does not take into account any lateral forces (membranal forces) or capillary forces.

The tonometry has two principal methods: digital tonometry and tonometry by instruments. The digital tonometry is a subjective method due to the intervention of physician fingers. There is no theory supporting this method. The tonometry by instruments is divided according to the instrument: applanation tonometry and indentation tonometry.

Measurements by applanation tonometry and indentation tonometry have influence of age, ametropies, geometrical parameters (CH, CCT, ECR, ICR), and corneal material parameters (E). Those factors influence in the amount of force necessary to produce the applanation of the corneal surface that is in touch with the tonometer applanation cone. This information was considered in a very broad manner to design the tonometry devices and their procedures; that is why these devices preserve some inaccuracies.

The applanation tonometry is a technique studied and perfectioned by Goldmann [31]. The instrument developed by Goldmann is based on the Imbert–Fick law. This law applied the Fick–Maklakoff principle that corresponds to the same definition for engineering pressure (Pressure = Force/Surface). It is mounted on the slit lamp used by ophthalmologists. Goldmann used the Imbert law through the application of a variable force over a constant applanation area (diameter of 3.06 mm); this area is formed while the instrument touches the patient's cornea.

The contact tonometer tip has a PMMA lens where there is a well-known circumscribed circular area; it is necessary to push the tonometer against the cornea to match this area with a flattened cornea. When this area is reached, the ophthalmologist makes a read of the apparatus related to the force necessary to flatten the cornea so it is possible to reach that preestablished area; $IOP = F/A$, where F is the force applied and A is the well-known area.

Barraquer [33] pointed out that where the IOP is measured through applanation tonometry, the applied force is variable, the flattened corneal surface is constant, and there is a minor displacement of volume of liquid.

In order to analyze all the forces participating in the applanation tonometry, it is important to consider that the cornea has an elastic force that rejects the applanation (N) and a lacrimal meniscus between the flat surface of the tonometer and the cornea, adhering the flattening surface to the cornea (Force M). This force needs to be added to the previous one as follows: $(P)(S) + N = F + M$, so $P = (F + M - N)/(S)$, where (P) is the intraocular pressure, (S) is the flattened surface, (F) is the force applied in the tonometer, and (M) is the force in the meniscus [34].

1.2 Geometrical and Functional Parameters for Tonometry

The "calibrated dimensions" is the term used for all the geometrical characteristics for the human cornea and the applanation zone for the contact tonometer measurement. The calibrated dimensions are ECR of 7.80 mm, CCT of 0.520 mm, and flattened area of 7.35 mm^2 [13]; according to Goldmann, any variation of these parameters will incur in a wrong measure for the IOP. The elasticity of the cornea was not considered for the development of the device (tonometers). The cornea was considered as an elastic membrane with an insignificant thickness.

1.3 Tonometry Devices (Indirect Measurement of IOP)

The tonometry has grown since the last 20 years. The former devices were based on mechanical actions, and, now, the tonometry is turning to a new kind of device directed to diminish the effects of flat areas, thick corneas, pain during the exam, covering of all ages, etc. If the reader wants a deeper study about tonometric devices, descriptions of all kind of devices are found on literature [3, 35, 36]. In the following paragraphs you will find a description of each device known until now.

1.3.1 The Goldmann Tonometer

Among several methodologies to determine the intraocular pressure (IOP), both invasive and noninvasive technologies, the Goldmann tonometry is considered the "gold standard" for this measurement as it is identified as the benchmark or reference pattern for any other measure determined as IOP.

During IOP measurement with the Goldmann tonometer (contact tonometer), it is necessary to highlight that the PMMA tip of the tonometer (Fig. 6.2) pushes the cornea (anterior-posterior movement) mechanically to generate a flat circular area on it (Fig. 6.3). The circular applanated surface corresponds to a circle of 3.06 mm of diameter. The procedure uses fluorescein to improve vision of contact area. If the fluorescein meniscus around the applanated area has a thickness of 1.80 mm (using the slit lamp with a zoom of × 10), M and N forces are supposed to be in equilibrium [34].

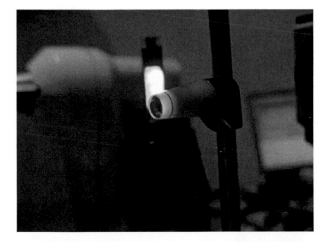

Fig. 6.2 The Goldmann tonometer slit lamp (*source*: Wikimedia Commons)

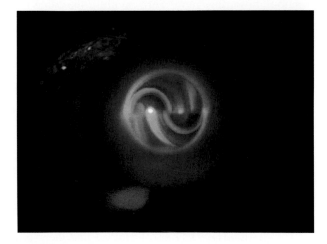

Fig. 6.3 Goldmann semicircles during tonometry (*source*: Wikimedia Commons)

According to Goldmann, the force needed to applanate the cornea (measured in grams) should be multiplied by 10 to measure IOP in mmHg.

When volume changes were checked inside the anterior chamber (and its influence on the IOP measurement), it results that there is no an important change (0.44 mm^3) [1]. That is why it is considered that the IOP = IOPt (pressure measured by the tonometer). Stamper et al. [37] explained that pressure difference between IOP and IOPt due to volumetric changes is 3 % (IOPt > IOP). Woo et al. [38] developed a curve relating IOP vs. ocular volume changes; this curve showed that little changes in volume, expressed in microliters, generate little IOP variations for pressure values lesser than 20 mmHg [38].

Due to all these mechanisms, from the engineering analysis, it is relevant to consider corneal parameters as the elasticity modulus (considering the cornea as an elastic material) or stress–strain curves that define the mechanical behavior of the cornea for the applanation procedure. Also, it will be relevant to know the Poisson ratio for compressibility analysis and the geometrical parameters of the cornea (ECR, ICR, CCT, LCT, etc.).

According to the previous arguments, it is necessary to point out that this device and the theory behind it have certain limitations. This device should be only applied on corneas with specific geometries. In addition, due to the device was set according to human adult corneas, it is questionable its usage on children or elderly patients.

The Goldmann tonometer consists in a dynamometer mounted in a system that allows to work with both the ophthalmic slit lamp and the ophthalmic microscope. The object that contacts the cornea is the applanation cone. The cone is mounted in the arm connected to the dynamometer). At the cone tip (contact zone) there is an embedded lens (measuring prism), manufactured in PMMA (E $= 3.00$ GPa, $\nu = 0.45$); over this lens there are several prismatic lenses that help to establish the exact applanation area corresponding to a diameter of two semi-rings of diameter of 3.06 mm each (total width for the tonometer tip is 7 mm; the contact zone is less than half of this diameter).

For the Goldmann tonometer, it is considered that the desired area of applanation is reached if the semi-rings get in touch in their inner portion at the off-center position (those rings move horizontally if the force is lowered or elevated). After the applanation area is reached, the reading of the dial in grams is multiplied by 10 to obtain the IOP in mmHg. The dial is aside the protective case for the dynamometer of the tonometer [37].

1.3.2 Pneumatic Tonometers (Pneumotonometer or PT)

This kind of tonometer changes the mechanical action for compressed gas. This is a portable device to measure the IOP.

Abbasoglu et al. [39] compared measures between the PT and the GAT. These measures were obtained after a PRK (photorefractive keratectomy). They found that the PT measures the IOP with confidence in each and every portion of the cornea after this procedure while the GAT underestimates the IOP in 2.40 ± 1.23 mmHg. They also identified that there is no influence of the CCT or the corneal irregularities on the measurement of IOP by means of the PT.

1.3.3   Rebound Tonometers

These tonometers eject a probe against the cornea (actio–reactio law). The probe is made with plastic, but it has a conductor material; the conductivity is necessary to eject the probe and to measure the movement in and out the tonometer. The IOP is determined due to the change of voltage induced in the probe movement. It was designed for a fast exam; any anesthetic or preparation is not necessary (Fig. 6.4).

1.3.4   Others

- *Pascal dynamic contour tonometer* (DCT): The DCT is an applanation tonometer that adapts to the corneal curvature. This device is portable (Fig. 6.5).

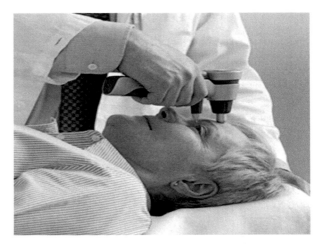

Fig. 6.4 I-Care rebound tonometer (adapted from www.icaretonometer.com)

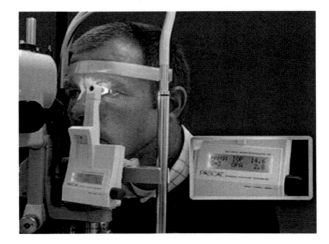

Fig. 6.5 Exam using the Pascal dynamic contour tonometer (*Source*: Wikimedia Commons)

Fig. 6.6 Exam using
Diaton transpalpebral
tonometer (*Source*:
Wikimedia Commons)

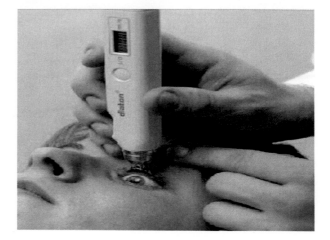

Kniestedt [40] and Kotecha et al. [25] identified that the DCT and the pneumotonometer showed less dependency on CCT related to the GAT measures.

- *Reichert's ocular response analyzer* (ORA): This device reports information about the corneal hysteresis; this is an additional biomechanical parameter to consider due to the impact of the mechanics of the tissue and its independence related to the corneal geometry.

  Lanza et al. [41] concluded in their research that the DCT or the ORA will be in the future the standard for tonometry due to their independence in the geometrical parameters that affects the Goldmann tonometry and its coherence with manometric measurements [42].

- *Diaton tonometer*: The Diaton tonometer measures IOP through the eyelid and with no damage to the cornea. It is portable and easy to use (Fig. 6.6). There are reports comparing its results against the GAT and other devices.

- *Tonopen*

2   Direct Measurement of IOP: Experimental Research

Experimentation is an important task in research activities. This activity relates the biomechanical behavior of the biological tissues with their material theoretical models. A proper characterization ensures an analytical model for certain procedures o extreme conditions during surgery.

For the tonometry, there are two types of experimentation: tensile tests or inflation of corneal buttons to determine the material properties for the cornea and sclera, and direct IOP tests by manometry.

2.1 Research in Animals

Due to the difficulty to find human tissues to perform mechanical tests, some researchers performed tests on animals to compare their mechanical properties with the corresponding of the humans.

Zeng et al. [43] performed tests on porcine corneas. They found that the average elasticity modulus for the porcine corneas is almost the same of the elasticity modulus for the human cornea (3.81 vs. 3.70 MPa).

DiSilvestro and Suh [44] compared three methodologies to validate a biphasic poroelastic model (BPVE: biphasic poro-visco-elastic model) in articular cartilage. They performed tests such as unconfined compression, indenting, and confined compression. Each prediction was performed through material parameters obtained from fitting curves of unconfined compression tests. The protocol for the tests includes a preparation of samples with pre-stretching of 10 % of the original length. This preparation assures that the tissue is ready to behave as a linear material.

Since the decade of 1960 leporids have been widely used for experimentation in ophthalmology [34, 45–47]. This experimentation developed through the determination of the true IOP by manometry. Sears [45] performed several manometry tests on sedated rabbits while the IOP was altered by different means (e.g., tearing of the iris).

Iinuma et al. [46] plotted the changes on IOP due to a constant load over the rabbit cornea. This kind of research has the objective to recreate the tonometric conditions. This work performed tests on rabbits and enucleated eyes from humans. The relevance of this research implies that give answer to incongruences for IOP determined with manometry. The manometry has several sources of error like the place where the eye is cannulated, the fluids and equipment used.

2.2 Research in Human Eye

Tensile tests and pressure test are the preferred tests in human eyes. Below, there is a review of documentation related to these tests and the computational models developed to understand the structural behavior of living tissues like the cornea. Non-linear behavior of these tissues make difficult the validation of these computational models.

3 Biomechanical Models of the Eye for Tonometry

Several researchers had performed tests on ocular tissues to report corneal mechanical behavior (stress–strain curves). The most important are uniaxial tensile strength test and inflation test in corneal buttons. For tonometry, applanation and indentation tests are of special interest to determine corneal rigidity not for membrane but for transversal loads.

Friedenwald was the first researcher that correlates the geometrical parameters for the eye with a "rigidity" coefficient [48, 49]. He designed a "plethysmographic" camera. This camera was able to detect changes of fluid volume in the anterior chamber due to corneal applanation. He also documented the influence of this procedure on the iris and the ciliary processes. To accomplish this, he replaced a known amount of aqueous humor for a gas bubble; for each test, while a tonometry measurement is performed, there is an extraction of a little amount of gas. This test is repeated along a timescale. Friedenwald concluded that a high rigidity is found in an eye with a low curvature radius (a flat eye suffers higher strains). He also established a calibration scale for the Goldmann tonometer. All his tests were performed in pig eyes, cat eyes, and rabbit eyes.

Schwartz et al. [50] determined the elasticity modulus for the epithelium. They studied the mechanical influence of this layer on applanation tonometry.

Some researchers as Armaly [51], McEwen [52], and Kronfeld [53] found that the corneal rigidity diminishes as IOP is increased. This statement was reevaluated by Orssengo and Pye [13] several years after.

Greene [54] performed inflation tests with cornea buttons. This study tried to find the mechanical properties of the cornea, specifically for epithelium and endothelium and their influence on the myopic refractive illness. He concluded that neither epithelium nor endothelium had any responsibility on corneal mechanics.

The mechanical properties for the cornea in compression were studied by Battaglioli and Kamm [55]. They found that the elasticity modulus for the cornea loaded in a radial direction was one hundred times smaller than the elasticity modulus for the membrane situation (circumferential stresses). The Poisson ratio was reported to vary from 0.46 to 0.50. Compression tests were performed in small cylindrical sections submitted to a compressive load of 200 Pa; after a stabilization time of 30 min, force and strain were measured (Fig. 6.7).

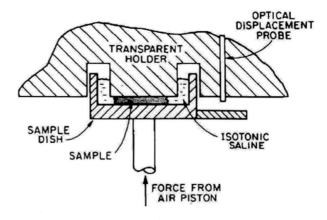

Fig. 6.7 Section cut for the positioner of the scleral sample in compression tests (adapted from Battaglioli and Kamm [55])

Fig. 6.8 Corneal layers.
Section cut: (**1**) epithelium,
(**2**) Bowman's membrane,
(**3**) stroma, (**4**) Descemet's
membrane, and (**5**)
endothelium (adapted
from [57])

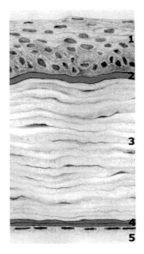

Figure 6.8 shows a section cut for the positioner of the scleral sample in compression tests (Adapted from Battaglioli and Kamm [55]).

In the following sections, we will present some analytical models for the corneal behavior accepted for tonometry.

3.1 Analytic Models to Represent the Corneal Material Behavior

For computational modeling, some authors [56] take into account the five layers for the cornea: endothelium, Descemet's membrane, stroma, Bowman's membrane, and epithelium (Fig. 6.8). Nevertheless, is widely accepted that the stroma is the main structure; it covers 90 % of the CCT (500 μm). The stroma is composed for collagen lamellae, ground substance, and keratocytes.

It is important to highlight that Bryant and McDonnell [58] developed models through finite element modeling with the objective to study the response of the cornea in the radial keratotomy. They developed three different models for each material considered: linear elastic isotropy, transversal linear elastic isotropy, and nonlinear isotropy. The geometric model considered was axisymmetric with mapped mesh. The mechanical properties for the material were obtained by experimentation with membrane inflation (human cornea buttons) and its comparison with nonlinear models with finite element analysis (Fig. 6.9). For linear models, the elasticity modulus varies from 0.79 to 0.83 MPa.

In the same work, Bryant and McDonnell recalled some results from previous studies in regard to determining the elasticity modulus for the cornea: 0.025 MPa [59] for IOP of 10.0 mmHg and 17.0 MPa [60] for IOP of 100 mmHg. They concluded that the corneal stiffness increases at higher pressures. This observation is evident in the experimental curves for pressure displacement in Fig. 6.9.

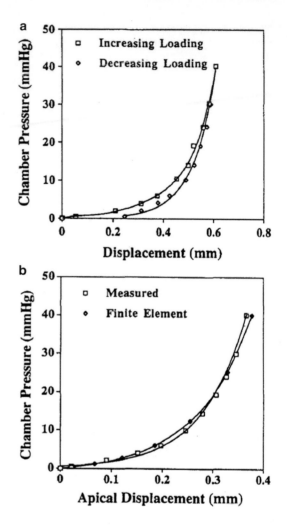

Fig. 6.9 (**A**, **B**). Curves for inflation tests for human cornea (adapted from Bryant and McDonnell [58])

Wang et al. [61] developed a technique to obtain the mechanical properties of the cornea through ultrasound. The samples of corneal strips were prepared with saline and dextran. The elasticity modulus for each preparation was 5.30 ± 1.1 MPa and 20.0 ± 0.1 MPa, respectively. The latter is similar to results for tensile tests reported for authors as Arciniegas and Amaya [4]. Wang et al. pointed out the causes of lack of consensus for the mechanical properties of the cornea:

- Nonlinearity of the mechanical properties for the cornea: stress–strain curves
- Quality of tissues: old tissues, altered tissues, or bad preservation of tissues
- Test method: inflation tests and tensile tests

3.1.1   Linear Models

The elastic behavior is present in most of the structural materials. They are characterized by a linear proportion between stress and strain for the material. For many phenomena associated with corneal pathologies, it is considered an elastic behavior for the corneal material; nevertheless, there is no consensus about a modulus of elasticity for each individual (e.g., according to age). This supposition is valid, while certain conditions are accomplished: corneal deformation and load type.

For tonometry, where it is important to establish the relevance of each influential parameter, it is considered appropriate to employ a linear elastic model due to the short-term process and the low deformation determined as elastic.

Mow [19] developed the "sandwich shell theory" aiming to estimate and analyze the mechanical properties for the elastic cornea during applanation tonometry. This theory includes several assumptions as considering three layers in the cornea with linear mechanic behavior. Mow concludes that his theory could be applied to applanation tonometry because the displacements induced by the tonometer are small enough to consider the cornea as a linear elastic material.

Amaya y Arciniegas [62] performed several experiments (tensile tests on corneal and scleral tissues) to calculate the stiffness of the eye globe tissues (average elasticity modulus for adult human cornea and sclera, $E = 20.0$ MPa). They performed these experiments for high levels of load and deformation (yield stress for human cornea and sclera: 4.00 MPa). They concluded that stiffness decays with age (Fig. 6.10). Some of these arguments have been controverted nowadays;

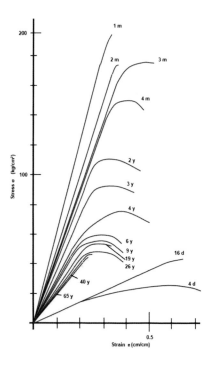

Fig. 6.10 Stress–strain curves vs. age. Experimentation in human sclera [62]

ElSheik et al. [7] demonstrated that stiffness is proportional to aging because of elastin loss. There is no consensus because there are no more conclusive reports; nevertheless, it is clear that it is not correct to use solely one elasticity modulus for the whole world population; it changes with age.

Pinsky and Datye [63] propose a model for the cornea where the structural responsibility is assigned to the stroma. They based their theory on the stromal microstructure and explained that the human cornea has flexural and shear rigidities that are insignificant compared with membrane rigidity. They proposed a biostructural model for the cornea as a thick shell where the tensile forces are resisted by collagen fibers embedded on the cell matrix. They consider a linear elastic model without time dependence.

Buzard [64] performed inflation tests to determine the elasticity modulus for the cornea. He found that secant elastic modulus is 7.58 MPa (constant) for IOP ranging from 25.0 to 100 mmHg.

Through ultrasound, it is possible to evaluate the particles' vibration on the cornea [61]. Wang et al. considered that the cornea can be considered as a lineal material in a specific deformational state due to the low vibration perceived on the ocular tissues.

Anderson et al. [65] suggest in their work that it is possible to consider the cornea as a linear elastic material if the IOP ranges from 15.0 to 30.0 mmHg. The elastic parameters used for their modeling are referred to Orssengo and Pye [13]: $E = 0.0229 \times IOP$ and $\nu = 0.49$. Dupps and Wilson [66] also recommend to use a Poisson ratio of 0.49 for biological tissues due to its noncompressibility condition and a solid matrix filled with fluid.

Hamilton and Pye [27] presented in their work that the elasticity modulus for a number of healthy young eyes is 0.29 ± 0.06 MPa. They performed a work where the Orssengo and Pye algorithm [13] is implemented and compared with experimental tests. The Poisson ratio was considered as 0.49. The authors stated that the IOP could be underestimated when the tonometry exam is performed in a cornea with a thick CCT due to its highly hydration. According to previous works [13, 18, 24, 27, 35, 59, 61, 67, 68] the elasticity modulus for the cornea varies from 0.10 to 57.0 MPa due to possible variation on tests conditions (there is no consensus about a standardized test). Authors also stated that the correction algorithms for the Goldmann tonometry that are based on CCT (solely) are incurring on errors for IOP estimation.

3.1.2 Multi-lineal Models

Kobayashi and Woo [69] made an important assumption that was implemented for the analysis of applanation tonometry. They stated that the corneal and scleral shells behave as an isotropic material when they are loaded on their situation of double curvature. The materials defined on this work are modulus of elasticity for stroma ($E = 2.0 \times 10^7$ dyna/cm^2 = 2.0 MPa), modulus of elasticity for sclera and for Descemet's membrane ($E = 5.5 \times 10^7$ dyna/cm^2 = 5.5 MPa), and Poisson ratio (0.45). Nyquist's research [70] was the source for some assumptions of this analytical study. Tonometry model developed by Kobayashi and Woo is depicted in Fig. 6.11.

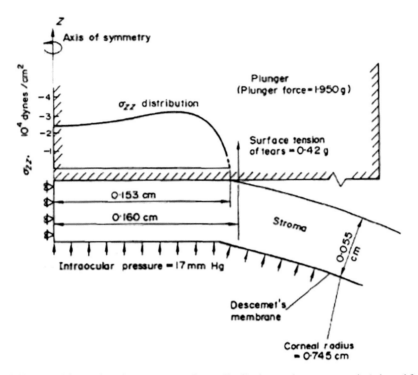

Fig. 6.11 Model for applanation tonometry. Stress distribution on the tonometer tip (adapted from Kobayashi and Woo [69])

One year later, Woo and Kobayashi [38] presented new information in regard to theories for modeling of corneal phenomena. Woo and Kobayashi assumed a modulus of elasticity for the corneal stroma of 2.0×10^5 dyna/cm^2 (20 kPa) during the applanation tonometry; this modulus coincides with approximations performed by Goldmann [71] for this modulus.

Woo and Kobayashi [72] also developed a trilinear model for corneal material (Fig. 6.12). These models were developed through tests on pressurized corneal buttons of human eyes enucleated 1–3 days after donor decease. For the modeling of applanation tonometry for physiological conditions of IOP, there were considered the elasticity modulus for the flatten stroma (loading condition for the tonometry) combined with the trilinear model [38]. Surface tension due to lacrimal film is considered in this work as 0.42 g for a corneal diameter of 3.20 mm [50]. They suggest for the first time to use a solid filled with fluid for tonometric modeling (poroelastic model).

It is believed that the most accurate procedure to determine the mechanical properties of the cornea is through inflation tests. This procedure has a strong similarity with corneal state in situ. Bryant and McDonnell [58] performed inflation tests in intact and fresh human corneas. They found that nonlinear corneal behavior is connected with a material nonlinearity (not geometrical).

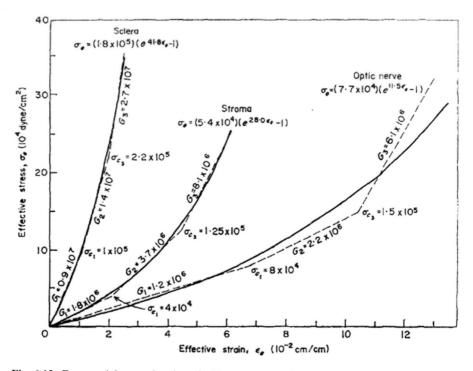

Fig. 6.12 Exponential approximation of trilinear stress–strain curves for ocular tissues (adapted from Woo and Kobayashi [72])

Modeling the cornea through the finite element method allows to infer that the transverse linear isotropy is not capable to model the anisotropy that had been evidenced during tests. Also, a hyperelastic law does not fit to the rigid behavior of the cornea. They considered the Poisson ratio as 0.49. To build a model with a transverse isotropy, it is possible to conclude that the elasticity modulus through the corneal thickness is ten times lesser than the elasticity modulus on the plane.

3.1.3 Nonlinear, Viscoelastic, and Biphasic (Poroelastic) Models

The biologic materials are different from the rest of materials used in engineering. These materials (biologic ones) are characterized by phenomena as creep (or deformation through time) and stress relaxation. This phenomenon is related to the variation on time of load of deformation. If this behavior is implemented in a computational model, it will be more accurate.

It should be noted that the stroma, the bigger layer for the cornea, is composed of water (78 % in weight), collagen fibers (15 % wt.), and proteins, proteoglycans, and salts (7 % wt.). This composition rules the mechanical behavior for the cornea [73].

As stated in 3.1.2, Woo and Kobayashi pointed out the necessity to consider a fluid inside the solid structure of the cornea.

Vito and Carnell [74], as other researchers, also considered to model the cornea including several layers especially during tonometry. They assumed that each layer is free to slide one against other. Also, they consider large displacements (combined with rigidity changes). As a result of their work, they recommend to increase the study of boundary conditions for tonometry because of its effects on both stress and strain. As most of the soft tissues, the cornea is considered as nonlinear and viscoelastic. Nevertheless, it is possible to obtain a good approximation of tonometry with a linear model with a modulus of elasticity for the cornea of $E = 2.00$ MPa and for the sclera of $E = 5.00$ MPa.

The material properties for the biological tissues are modeled as poroelastic models constituted by two phases: solid and fluid. Also, these tissues are subjected to finite deformations during normal daily activities and in the physiological range [75]. About this research, it is highlighted that opposite to many porous materials in engineering, hydrated biological tissues overcome great deformations in short periods. These deformations occur during lab test conditions where it is difficult to represent the physiological conditions (loads and restraints) for the eye globe.

In the same work, Levenston et al. performed a simplified version of the theory and formulation of biphasic modeling. They also addressed several variational formulations for the biphasic problem (Lagrange multiplier form, penalty form, and augmented Lagrangian form); after that, they presented the finite element implementation and its description with numerical examples.

In the computational modeling of the cornea, where it is required that the material should be treated as viscoelastic, it is necessary to have information about the permeability of each corneal layer. Prausnitz and Noonan [76] published information about permeability of each layer for the cornea against different kind of medicines regarding to evaluate the effectiveness in drug delivery. These permeability values (in animals) are summarized as referent:

– Minimum: 1.0×10^{-7} cm/s
– Maximum: $1.0 \times 10^{-3.5}$ cm/s
– Average: 1.0×10^{-5} cm/s

Other values of permeability for the cornea to study drug delivery and through different methods could be found in literature [77–81].

Through tensile tests in porcine eyes [43], it is possible to conclude that the mechanical models for porcine cornea are not suitable for research in human corneas where viscoelastic phenomena should be considered. Both corneas have different behavior on time; both corneas have different mechanical properties and different fluxes inside and outside the cornea.

In the work of Katsube et al. [82] is presented a solid model filled with fluid. In their work, the authors explain why the intact cornea has a strong tendency to absorb water to regularize its normal function. They also explained the behavior of water inside the living cornea and its function to maintain a negative pressure (sub-atmospheric pressure; 50–60 mmHg below the atmospheric pressure). This negative pressure is called imbibition pressure. The swelling property of the cornea can change through corneal thickness due to several bio-chemical regions with different hydration properties.

Ethier et al. [35] presented a revision of the literature according to average values for the elasticity modulus of the corneoscleral shell. They stated a range of 5.00–13.0 MPa. In their research, they presented an explanation of the developed theories to explain the behavior of the corneoscleral material, including the biphasic theory; this theory takes importance due to the time-dependent behavior of the cornea (viscoelastic material). This description evokes the heterogeneity of the cornea and its highly anisotropic behavior including its nonlinearity.

Another contribution of Ethier et al. [35] was a development of an equation that represents the viscoelastic behavior for the cornea. This equation was derived from the stress relaxation technique (time dependent) on corneoscleral strips.

$$y = -0.0159 \ln(t) + 0.9785 \tag{6.11}$$

The simplest formulation for viscoelasticity is to consider a biphasic model for the cornea. To achieve this goal, it is necessary to perform formulations that set the coupling between solid and liquid phases composing the tissue. Prokofiev and Dunec [83] presented a simple methodology for poroelastic formulation in COMSOL package. This formulation coincides with the formulation presented at Rémond et al. [84].

In poroelastic biphasic models, where it is considered the interstitial fluid, it is important to consider the barriers present in the cornea and the proper actions for its maintenance. This subject was treated by Dupps and Wilson [66]; they describe specific characteristics of the human cornea as: hydrophilic characteristic of the stromal glycosaminoglycans [85], imbibition pressure, corneal hydration level [86], stromal swelling pressure, and active endothelial transport [87].

The cornea is a complex anisotropic compound with nonlinear elastic properties including viscoelasticity [66] (Fig. 6.13). Dupps and Wilson refer that interlamellar shear strength is weaker than the corneal tensile strength; this situation grants the

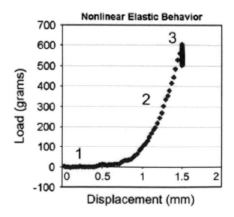

Fig. 6.13 Nonlinear elastic properties for a corneal strip of 7 mm; 63-year-old patient (with permission of Dupps and Wilson [66])

corneal stability and the mainly tensile stress state. They also identified that just the corneal stroma and Bowman's membrane have collagen fibers (responsible of tensile strength); also, they found that Bowman's membrane removal doesn't affect the mechanical properties of the cornea (agreeing with [88]). This latter finding was possible through tensile tests and stress relaxation tests for corneal strips (Fig. 6.14).

4   Computational Modeling for the Applanation Tonometry

From the biomechanics, the eye is a pressure vessel with structural walls called the cornea and sclera. This vessel is called ophthalmoid (term minted for Arciniegas and Amaya [89]; two spheroids joined by a transition surface) (Fig. 6.15). Inside the vessel, it is possible to find several nonstructural elements: the iris, lens, ciliary zonule, ciliary body, and retina (Fig. 6.16). The ophthalmoid keeps its shape due to the internal pressure (IOP) produced by the aqueous and vitreous humors (Fig. 6.17). The eye globe is suspended by a group of muscles that restraint its movements in the axial (anterior-posterior) and rotational directions [89].

It has been shown that there are different components inside the cornea with specific responsibilities for mechanical resistance. Mechanical tests on soft tissues help to understand that the collagen and elastin fibers exhibit a great tensile

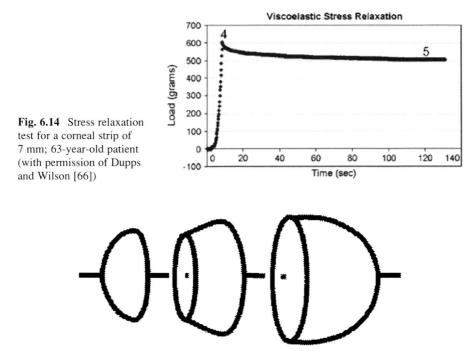

Fig. 6.14 Stress relaxation test for a corneal strip of 7 mm; 63-year-old patient (with permission of Dupps and Wilson [66])

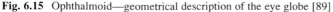

Fig. 6.15 Ophthalmoid—geometrical description of the eye globe [89]

Fig. 6.16 Eye globe
anatomy (adapted
from [35])

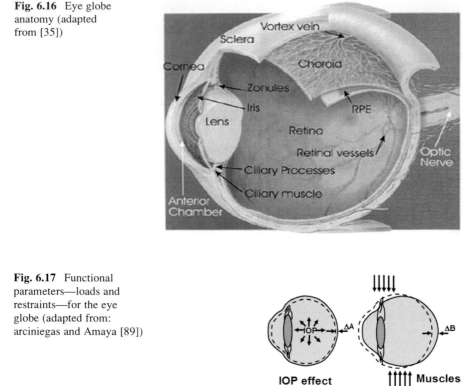

Fig. 6.17 Functional
parameters—loads and
restraints—for the eye
globe (adapted from:
arciniegas and Amaya [89])

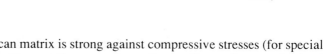

strength; the proteoglycan matrix is strong against compressive stresses (for special
interest in tonometry). For tensile tests, the collagen fibers align to the load
direction and then resist the load applied [90].

4.1   Finite Element Method in Corneal Biomechanics

One of the most relevant works in biomechanics is granted to Fung [91, 92]. Fung
performed several experiments with biological tissues (hard and soft tissues) as elongation and compression; he developed several stress–strain figures for biological tissues.

Bryant and McDonnell [58] established the material constitutive relationships
for the eye globe. They supposed that the cornea is incompressible (Poisson ratio of
0.49). In the same work, they performed numerical models for the cornea in 2D.
The cornea was subjected to increments in IOP. Results were compared with tests
for inflated corneal buttons obtaining good correlation in the apical displacement.
The computational model was isotropic with nonlinear elastic material.

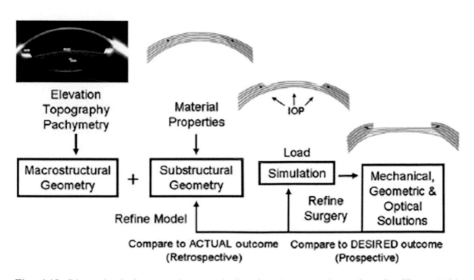

Elevation
Topography
Pachymetry

Material
Properties

IOP

Load

| Macrostructural Geometry | + | Substructural Geometry | | Simulation | → | Mechanical, Geometric & Optical Solutions |

Refine Model

Refine Surgery

Compare to ACTUAL outcome
(Retrospective)

Compare to DESIRED outcome
(Prospective)

Fig. 6.18 Biomechanical approach to analysis of ocular surgeries and ocular illness (with permission of Dupps and Wilson [66])

As established for Amaya and Arciniegas [34], the eye globe is considered as a pressure vessel with thin walls. The eye is a hollow body, is closed, and contains a fluid with a different pressure to the external pressure.

Anderson et al. [65] published a work about several applications of the structural engineering on the ophthalmology. They prepare a tridimensional model for the tonometry but no results were discussed.

In 2006, Dupps and Wilson [66] presented in their work about corneal biomechanics the stages that are included on corneal modeling through finite element method (Fig. 6.18). It can be identified three stages for data collection: macrostructural geometry (corneal height, corneal topography, pachymetry), substructural geometry (material properties), and boundary conditions (loads and restraints—IOP, muscles, corneal limbus). This methodology is applied for LASIK surgery simulation in a retrospective way (evaluating current clinical data) or in a prospective way (predicting results).

For biomechanical study of the eye it is necessary to identify three series of basic parameters: geometrical parameters, material parameters, and functional parameters.

4.1.1 Geometrical Parameters

These parameters include dimensions and exact curves for the vessel. For the eye globe: ECR, ICR, CCT, and corneal height (CH).

The eye globe has a nonuniform thickness along cornea walls; this thickness is almost constant for the scleral tissue except for the eye walls in the corneal limbus and optic head nerve root.

The ocular globe dimensions are, in average, 24 mm in medial-nasal direction (eye globe diameter). It is composed mainly by three layers (fibrous, vascular, and inner layers), the lens and two main cavities (anterior and posterior chamber) [41].

4.1.2 Material Parameters

Elastomechanic properties. For the eye globe: refractive index, Poisson ratio, elasticity modulus (Young modulus for linear elastic material), and allowable stresses for the material.

Chapter 3 includes a description about tests and findings in regard to corneal biomechanics.

4.1.3 Functional Parameters

Loads and restraints. For the eye globe: IOP and support conditions for the cornea (Fig. 6.17).

The human eye is a structure with several complex processes. It is composed by several elements and several differential functions that grant its stability, nutrition, transparency, and functionality.

The corneal and scleral microstructure has been studied by Woo et al. [72] and Hjortdal [94]. Their research has been directed to develop new methodologies to correct optic aberrations. Recent studies were redirected to study the effects of refractive surgeries due to the ignorance of the structural responsibility of each layer in the corneal tissue.

As Guyton and Hall [2] describe, the eye is filled by a fluid (aqueous and vitreous humor) that maintains enough pressure to distend the eye globe. The aqueous humor could be found between the anterior face of the lens and the posterior face of the cornea, and the vitreous humor could be found between the retina and the posterior face of the lens.

The aqueous humor is a fine and transparent fluid composed as the blood plasma. This liquid moves smoothly and freely inside the eye. The vitreous humor is a jelly mass that is held together between them by a net of fine fibers composed mainly by long proteoglycans molecules. The water and the dissolved substances can diffuse slowly in the vitreous, but this process is hard due to a reduced fluid flux. Entrance and exit channels are depicted in Fig. 6.19.

The aqueous humor is secreted by the ciliary processes. These processes are folded structures that project from the ciliary bodies to the space behind the iris where lens ligaments and the ciliary muscle get fixed to the eye globe; they have a surface area of 6 cm^2 by the eye. Below the ciliary processes there is a highly vascularized area; the aqueous humor is a product of high filtration of blood. The aqueous humor is formed and reabsorbed constantly; this controlled or balanced process regulates the total volume and the fluid pressure (IOP).

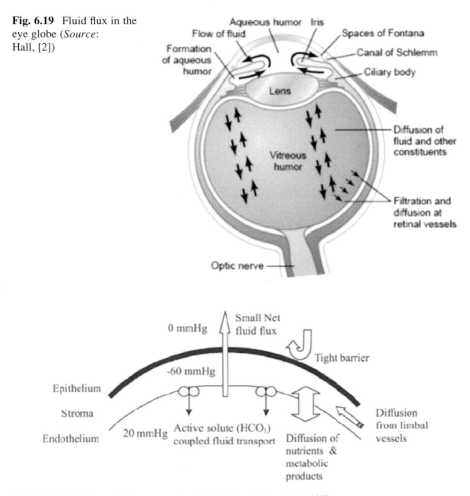

Fig. 6.19 Fluid flux in the eye globe (*Source*: Hall, [2])

Fig. 6.20 Flux through the cornea (reprinted from Ethier et al., [35])

The aqueous humor dynamics is described by Jones and Maurice [95], Sampaolesi [1], Wiig [96], Ethier et al. [35], and Hall [2]. Since the cornea does not have blood vessel for nutrition due to its transparency requirements, the aqueous humor is its source of nutrients. The rate of production of aqueous humor is 2.4 ± 0.6 µl/min (for adults between 20 and 83 years old). This rate has a diurnal variation; the highest is in the morning (3.0 µl/min), and the lowest is during the night (1.5 µl/min). The authors refer that there is an outwards flux velocity of 20 µm/h from inside the cornea to the lacrimal film; nevertheless, the corneal endothelium produces an inward flux velocity of 40 µm/h. The fluid flux produces changes of pressure inside the corneal stroma creating mechanic strains (compression). Figure 6.20 depicts the flux components inside the cornea.

Due to its interest in tonometry and its influence on aqueous humor dynamics, permeability of endothelium and epithelium was studied by Klyce and Rusell [97]. They report an analysis considering thermodynamics about flux on corneal endothelium; the permeability to water of endothelium is seven times higher than permeability on epithelium.

4.2 Assumptions for Computational Models for the Cornea

Most of the computational models for the cornea consider nonlinear material properties and geometries according to the cornea parameters. Boundary conditions are variable according if the model considers just the cornea or the entire globe (inflation tests).

A 2D model shows to be sufficient to explain deformational behavior to the tonometry process.

A 3D model with solid elements in three layers, employed for tonometry studies is shown in Fig. 6.21.

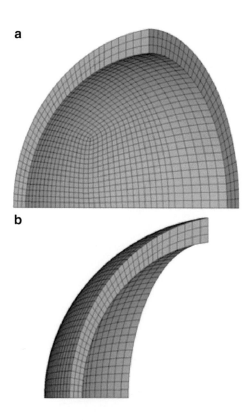

Fig. 6.21 (**A, B**)
Computational model for
the human cornea (posterior
and anterior view)

5 Tonometric Correction Equations for Applanation Tonometry

5.1 Problems with Applanation Tonometers

In the literature there are several arguments about problems regarding applanation tonometers based on the Imbert's law as the Goldmann tonometer [15, 21, 22, 24, 26, 27, 34, 57].

- The cornea is not a homogenous membrane. It is not infinitely thin. The CCT plays a main role in the measure of the IOP due to evidences as the higher measures of IOP obtained in thicker corneas.
- The cornea is not an elastic membrane. This is a valid approach for small deformations. There is no consensus about the corneal rigidity values (linear elasticity modulus for the physiological range of deformations).
- There are differences between the applanation area in the anterior and posterior faces for the cornea. This is due to the CCT.
- During applanation tonometry, there is a displacement of the aqueous humor. In addition, there is a relaxing behavior of the sclerotic tissue and an increment of the IOP, producing a variable volume of fluid. All these mechanisms depend on corneal curvature.
- The surface tension of the precorneal tear film and the liquid ring formed around the applanated circle (between the cornea and the flattened surface) create additional adhesion forces (capillary forces).
- The tonometric measurement is difficult for astigmatic corneas.
- Aging affects the geometrical properties and material mechanical properties for the cornea. Aging affects the tonometric measure due to its dependence on these parameters.
- The tonometric measures are different between races and communities. Some ethnical groups have more or less CCT compared with others.
- There are mistakes on mathematical foundation for tonometric interpretation. According to Friedenwald [48], the mathematical equation that represents the linearized curve for his graphic analysis is: $(dP/P) = k \, (dV/V)$. This equation represents a straight line with intercept in the origin. This equation does not take into account the logarithm for the pressure to linearize this curve. Regardless of this mistake on this equation, there are still references on the literature citing to the Friedenwald's constant called "K" and its theory [98–101].
- Consecutive measurements of the IOP incur in mistakes due to the viscoelastic behavior of the cornea (creep and stress relaxation properties). The effect is an underestimation of the value (reduced values).

Due to these problems, it is necessary to consider tonometric correction equations for the applanation tonometry.

5.2 Tonometric Correction Equations

Some reviews about different approaches for calibration equations could be found on the literature [12, 13, 15, 17, 18, 22, 23, 40, 102–106]. Some of them take into account the CCT solely. This approach of a uniparametric equation has been reevaluated; new equations consider biomechanical parameters (elasticity modulus) and geometrical parameters (ECR and CCT) for the cornea.

It is important to note that each calibration equation is specifically designed for certain patient condition (normal, glaucomatous, post-LASIK) and for a range of parameters (ECR, CCT, age, biomechanical parameters—they change with age). There is not a generic equation for all devices or conditions. That is why, it is said that a new tonometric device will take the position of "Gold Standard" in the sense that it should be capable of capture less noise that could affect its measure (reliability).

Some tonometric correction equations for the GAT and their assumptions are described in Table 6.1.

Table 6.1 GAT correction equations (adapted from Chihara [15])

Author	Año	Equation	Comments
Ehlers et al. [12]	1975	$IOPT = \frac{IOPG - b}{0.561 + 0.000781 \times CCT}$	b is experimentally determined
Whitacre et al. [22]	1993	$IOPT = IOPG + 12.28 - (0.02283 \times CCT)$ $IOPT = IOPG + 22.38 - (0.04644 \times CCT)$	CCT < 0.52 mm
Orssengo and Pye [13]	1999	$IOPT = \dfrac{IOPG}{\left(\frac{42.4 \times CCT^2}{10^4 \times A(\mu)(ECR \times 10^3 - CCT/2)} + \frac{3.97 \times (ECR \times 10^3 - CCT/2) \times CCT}{A(\mu) \times 10^8} \right)}$	$A(\mu)$ varies with ECR and CCT
Foster et al. [103]	2000	$IOPT = 1.08 \times IOPG + 5.5$ mmHg	–
Feltgen et al. [23]	2001	$IOPT = IOPG + 3.43$ mmHg	–
Shimmyo et al. [104]	2003	$IOPT = IOPG + \frac{(550 - CCT)}{18 e^{-0.005 IOPG} + 0.8(ECR - 7.848837)}$	–
Kniestedt [40]	2005	$IOPT = IOPG + 3.43 \pm 1.24$ mmHg (nonlinear)	The CCT vs. IOPG slope change at CCT: 535 µm
Kohlhaas [106]	2006	$IOPT = IOPG + 23.28 - (0.0423 \times CCT)$	–
Chihara [15]	2008	$IOPT = \dfrac{IOPG + 4.15}{\left(\frac{19.99 \times CCT^2}{A(\mu) \times (ECR \times 10^3 - CCT/2) \times 10^4} + 1 \right)}$	$A(\mu)$ varies with ECR and CCT
Elsheikh et al [17]	2011	$IOPT = (-0.0372 \times Age) + (28.192 \times CCT)$ $+ (-1.556 \times ECR) + 26.707$	Age > 50 years
Guzmán et al. [18]	2013	$IOPT = (IOPG \times 1.59) + (0.931 \times ECR) -$ $(30.4 \times CCT)$	ECR: 7.60–7.90 mm, CCT: 0.510– 0.550 mm)

Conclusion

From biomechanics, if corneal thickness is considered as a fundamental part of rigidity against applanation, it can be stated that two corneas with the same geometry but different thicknesses will obtain different IOP measurements due to its necessity to apply a higher force in the thicker cornea to flatten the well-known area of the tonometer tip.

The same results will be obtained if it is considered a stepper cornea (highly myopic eye). This geometry will develop a higher rigidity against applanation. The Goldmann tonometer does not have these curvature variations among human eyes into account. It is important to consider that children's eyes are smaller than adult eyes, and it will influence IOP measurements. It is more difficult to flatten children corneas. It will incur in higher IOP measurements.

Due to new myopic LASIK surgeries, cases with lower IOPs had been reported. This change on IOP measurement can be attributed to the changes on the stromal layers and the reduced corneal thickness; LASIK surgery induced a curvature change (a higher radius), so it's easiest to flatten that cornea. It is necessary to perform research on these changes and check if this lowered IOP is constant in time or if this is a temporary condition.

Despite numerous research in biomechanics focused in ophthalmology and the understanding of biomechanical behavior of cornea, there is no unique model that explains each and every phenomena that occurs in daily practice for the ophthalmologists. Nevertheless, it is possible to perform simplified models that help to understand some phenomena with special detailings for each case.

Glossary

CCT Central corneal thickness
CH Corneal hysteresis, a measure of viscoelasticity of the cornea (elasticity)
CRF Corneal resistance factor
DCT Dynamic contour tonometer
E Linear elastic modulus (Young's modulus)
ECR External corneal radius
GAT Goldmann applanation tonometer
ICR Internal corneal radius
IOP Intraocular pressure
IOPcc IOP compensated for corneal effects
IOPg Goldmann equivalent IOP
IOPt Intraocular pressure measured by means of a tonometer
LCT Limbal corneal thickness

PR Poisson's ratio
PT Pneumotonometer
WS Waveform score

References

1. R. Sampaolesi, *Glaucoma* (Editorial Médica Panamericana S.A., Buenos Aires, 1974)
2. J.E. Hall, *Guyton and Hall Textbook of Medical Physiology* (Saunders, Enhanced E-Book, 2010)
3. C. Kniestedt, O. Punjabi, S. Lin, R.L. Stamper, Tonometry through the ages. Surv. Ophthalmol. **53**(6), 568–591 (2008)
4. A. Arciniegas, L.E. Amaya, Mechanical behavior of the Sclera. Ophthalmologica **193**(1–2), 45–55 (1986)
5. P.-A. Tonnu, T. Ho, T. Newson, A. El Sheikh, K. Sharma, E. White et al., The influence of central corneal thickness and age on intraocular pressure measured by pneumotonometry, non-contact tonometry, the Tono-Pen XL, and Goldmann applanation tonometry. Br. J. Ophthalmol. **89**(7), 851–854 (2005)
6. A. Kotecha, A. Elsheikh, C.R. Roberts, H. Zhu, D.F. Garway-Heath, Corneal thickness- and age-related biomechanical properties of the cornea measured with the ocular response analyzer. Invest. Ophthalmol. Vis. Sci. **47**(12), 5337–5347 (2006)
7. A. Elsheikh, D. Wang, M. Brown, P. Rama, M. Campanelli, D. Pye, Assessment of corneal biomechanical properties and their variation with age. Curr. Eye Res. **32**(1), 11–19 (2007)
8. A. Elsheikh, D. Wang, P. Rama, M. Campanelli, D. Garway-Heath, Experimental assessment of human corneal hysteresis. Curr. Eye Res. **33**(3), 205–213 (2008)
9. T. Kida, J.H.K. Liu, R.N. Weinreb, Effects of aging on corneal biomechanical properties and their impact on 24-hour measurement of intraocular pressure. Am. J. Ophthalmol. **146**(4), 567–572.e1 (2008)
10. T. Gosho, K. Yamada, N. Yamasaki, M. Higashimori, J. Takenaka, Y. Kiuchi et al., Is cornea compliant with respect to age? in *World Congr. Med. Phys. Biomed. Eng. Sept. 7–12 2009 Munich Ger*, ed. by O. Dössel, W. Schlegel (Springer, Berlin, 2009), pp. 223–226
11. A. Elsheikh, B. Geraghty, P. Rama, M. Campanelli, K.M. Meek, Characterization of age-related variation in corneal biomechanical properties. J. R. Soc. Interface **7**(51), 1475–1485 (2010)
12. N. Ehlers, T. Bramsen, S. Sperling, Applanation tonometry and central corneal thickness. Acta Ophthalmol. (Copenh) **53**(1), 34–43 (1975)
13. G. Orssengo, D. Pye, Determination of the true intraocular pressure and modulus of elasticity of the human cornea in vivo. Bull. Math. Biol. **61**(3), 551–572 (1999)
14. M.E. Iliev, A. Meyenberg, E. Buerki, G. Shafranov, M.B. Shields, Novel pressure-to-cornea index in glaucoma. Br. J. Ophthalmol. **91**(10), 1364–1368 (2007)
15. E. Chihara, Assessment of true intraocular pressure: the gap between theory and practical data. Surv. Ophthalmol. **53**(3), 203–218 (2008)
16. T.H. Kwon, J. Ghaboussi, D.A. Pecknold, Y.M.A. Hashash, Effect of cornea material stiffness on measured intraocular pressure. J. Biomech. **41**(8), 1707–1713 (2008)
17. A. Elsheikh, D. Alhasso, P. Gunvant, D. Garway-Heath, Multiparameter correction equation for Goldmann applanation tonometry. Optom. Vis. Sci. **88**(1), E102–E112 (2011)
18. A.F. Guzmán, A. Arciniegas Castilla, F.A. Guarnieri, R.F. Ramírez, Intraocular pressure: Goldmann tonometry, computational model, and calibration equation. J. Glaucoma **22**(1), 10–14 (2013)
19. C.C. Mow, A theoretical model of the cornea for use in studies of tonometry. Bull. Math. Biophys. **30**(3), 437–453 (1968)

20. M. Whitacre, M. Emig, K. Hassanein, The effect of Perkins, Tono-Pen, and Schiotz tonometry on intraocular pressure. Am J. Ophthalmol. **111**(1), 59–64 (1991)
21. M.M. Whitacre, R. Stein, Sources of error with use of Goldmann-type tonometers. Surv. Ophthalmol. **38**(1), 1–30 (1993)
22. M. Whitacre, R. Stein, K. Hassanein, The effect of corneal thickness on applanation tonometry. Am J. Ophthalmol. **115**(5), 592–596 (1993)
23. N. Feltgen, D. Leifert, J. Funk, Correlation between central corneal thickness, applanation tonometry, and direct intracameral IOP readings. Br. J. Ophthalmol. **85**(1), 85–87 (2001)
24. J. Liu, C.J. Roberts, Influence of corneal biomechanical properties on intraocular pressure measurement: quantitative analysis. J. Cataract Refract. Surg. **31**(1), 146–155 (2005)
25. A. Kotecha, E.T. White, J.M. Shewry, D.F. Garway-Heath, The relative effects of corneal thickness and age on Goldmann applanation tonometry and dynamic contour tonometry. Br. J. Ophthalmol. **89**(12), 1572–1575 (2005)
26. A.T. Broman, N.G. Congdon, K. Bandeen-Roche, H.A. Quigley, Influence of corneal structure, corneal responsiveness, and other ocular parameters on tonometric measurement of intraocular pressure. J. Glaucoma **16**(7), 581–588 (2007)
27. K.E. Hamilton, D.C. Pye, Young's modulus in normal corneas and the effect on applanation tonometry. Optom. Vis. Sci. **85**(6), 445–450 (2008). doi:10.1097/OPX.0b013e3181783a70
28. H.H. Mark, Armand Imbert, Adolf Fick, and their tonometry law. Eye **26**(1), 13–16 (2012)
29. H. Goldmann, T. Schmidt, Über Applanationstonometrie. Ophthalmologica **134**(4), 221–242 (1957)
30. H. Goldmann, T. Schmidt, Weiterer Beitrag zur Applanationstonometrie. Ophthalmologica **141**(6), 441–456 (1961)
31. H. Goldmann, Un nouveau tonometre d'applanation. Bull. Soc. Ophtalmol. Fr **67**, 474–478 (1955)
32. G.C. Stuckey, Application of physical principles in the development of tonometry. Clin. Exp. Ophthalmol. **32**(6), 633–636 (2004)
33. J.I. Barraquer, *Cirugía refractiva de la córnea. LXV Ponen Soc Española Oftalmol* (Instituto Barraquer de América, Bogotá, 1989), pp. 812–814
34. A. Arciniegas, L.E. Amaya, Relación entre la tonometría de Goldmann y la presion intravitrea en conejos; Relation between the Goldmann tonometry and the intravitreous pressure in rabbits. Arch. Soc. Am. Oftalmol. Optom. **18**(4), 261–275 (1984)
35. C.R. Ethier, M. Johnson, J. Ruberti, Ocular biomechanics and biotransport. Annu. Rev. Biomed. Eng. **6**(1), 249–273 (2004)
36. M.K. ElMallah, S.G. Asrani, New ways to measure intraocular pressure. Curr. Opin. Ophthalmol. **19**(2), 122–126 (2008)
37. R.L. Stamper, M.F. Lieberman, M.V. Drake, Ch 4 – Intraocular pressure, in: *Becker-Shaffers Diagn. Ther. Glaucomas*, 8th edn. (Mosby, Edinburgh, 2009), pp. 47–67
38. S.L.-Y. Woo, A.S. Kobayashi, C. Lawrence, W.A. Schlegel, Mathematical model of the corneo-scleral shell as applied to intraocular pressure–volume relations and applanation tonometry. Ann. Biomed. Eng. **1**(1), 87–98 (1972)
39. Ö.E. Abbasolu, R.W. Bowman, H.D. Cavanagh, J.P. McCulley, Reliability of intraocular pressure measurements after myopic excimer photorefractive keratectomy. Ophthalmology **105**(12), 2193–2196 (1998)
40. C.L.S. Kniestedt, Clinical comparison of contour and applanation tonometry and their relationship to pachymetry. Arch. Ophthalmol. **123**(11), 1532–1537 (2005)
41. M. Lanza, M. Borrelli, M. De Bernardo, M.L. Filosa, N. Rosa, Corneal parameters and difference between Goldmann applanation tonometry and dynamic contour tonometry in normal eyes. J. Glaucoma **17**(6), 460–464 (2008)
42. A. Kotecha, What biomechanical properties of the cornea are relevant for the clinician? Surv. Ophthalmol. **52**(6, Supplement), S109–S114 (2007)
43. Y. Zeng, J. Yang, K. Huang, Z. Lee, X. Lee, A comparison of biomechanical properties between human and porcine cornea. J. Biomech. **34**(4), 533–537 (2001)

44. M.R. DiSilvestro, J.-K.F. Suh, A cross-validation of the biphasic poroviscoelastic model of articular cartilage in unconfined compression, indentation, and confined compression. J. Biomech. **34**(4), 519–525 (2001)
45. M.L. Sears, Miosis and intraocular pressure changes during manometry: mechanically irritated rabbit eyes studied with improved manometric technique. AMA Arch. Ophthalmol. **63**(4), 707–714 (1960)
46. I. Iinuma, K. Uenoyama, T. Sakaguchi, Intraocular pressure changes during tonography. Studies of other pressure tests in rabbit and enucleated human eyes by closed electric manometry. Am. J. Ophthalmol. **61**(5 Pt 1), 853–859 (1966)
47. P. Vareilles, P. Conquet, J.-C. Le Douarec, A method for the routine intraocular pressure (IOP) measurement in the rabbit: range of IOP variations in this species. Exp. Eye Res. **24**(4), 369–375 (1977)
48. J.S. Friedenwald, Contribution to the theory and practice of tonometry. Am J. Ophthalmol. **20** (9), 985–1024 (1937)
49. J.S. Friedenwald, H.F. Pierce, Circulation of the aqueous: VI. Intra-ocular gas exchange. Arch. Ophthalmol. **17**(3), 477–485 (1937)
50. N.J. Schwartz, R.S. Mackay, J.L. Sackman, A theoretical and experimental study of the mechanical behavior of the cornea with application to the measurement of intraocular pressure. Bull. Math. Biophys. **28**(4), 585–643 (1966)
51. M.F. Armaly, The heritable nature of dexamethasone-induced ocular hypertension. Arch. Ophthalmol. **75**(1), 32–35 (1966)
52. W.K. McEwen, Difficulties in measuring intraocular pressure and ocular rigidity, in *Glaucoma – Tultzing Symp Tultzing Castle,* ed by W. Leydhecker (1966), pp. 97–125
53. P. Kronfeld, Gross anatomy and embryology of the eye. The Eye **1**, 1–66 (1962)
54. P.R. Greene, Mechanical aspects of myopia, Ph.D. Thesis (Harvard University, Cambridge, 1978)
55. J.L. Battaglioli, R.D. Kamm, Measurements of the compressive properties of scleral tissue. Invest. Ophthalmol. Vis. Sci. **25**(1), 59–65 (1984)
56. N. Ehlers, J. Hjortdal, The cornea: epithelium and stroma, in *Adv. Organ Biol.* ed. by J. Fischbarg (Elsevier, Philadelphia, 2005), pp. 83–111
57. I. Asensio Romero, Valoración del efecto de la oxibuprocaína HCL 0.4 % y del compuesto de tetracaína y oxibuprocaína HCL 0.4 % sobre los valores anatómicos del espesor corneal humano. Ph.D. Thesis (Universitat de València, España, 2007)
58. M.R. Bryant, P.J. McDonnell, Constitutive laws for biomechanical modeling of refractive surgery. J. Biomech. Eng. **118**(4), 473–481 (1996)
59. E. Sjøntoft, C. Edmund, In vivo determination of young's modulus for the human cornea. Bull. Math. Biol. **49**(2), 217–232 (1987)
60. J.O. Hjortdal, P. Koch-Jensen, In situ mechanical behavior of the human cornea as evaluated by simultaneous measurement of corneal strain, corneal surface contour, and corneal thickness. Invest. Ophthalmol. Vis. Sci. **33**, 895 (1992)
61. H. Wang, P.L. Prendiville, P.J. McDonnell, W.V. Chang, An ultrasonic technique for the measurement of the elastic moduli of human cornea. J. Biomech. **29**(12), 1633–1636 (1996)
62. L.E. Amaya, A. Arcienegas, *Mecánica de la cavidad ocular* (Universidad de los Andes, Facultad de Ingeniería, Centro de Estudios e Investigación, Bogotá, 1982)
63. P.M. Pinsky, D.V. Datye, A microstructurally-based finite element model of the incised human cornea. J. Biomech. **24**(10), 907–922 (1991)
64. K. Buzard, Introduction to biomechanics of the cornea. Refract. Corneal. Surg. **8**(2), 127–138 (1992)
65. K. Anderson, A. El-Sheikh, T. Newson, Application of structural analysis to the mechanical behaviour of the cornea. J. R. Soc. Interface **1**(1), 3–15 (2004)
66. W.J. Dupps Jr., S.E. Wilson, Biomechanics and wound healing in the cornea. Exp. Eye Res. **83**(4), 709–720 (2006)

67. J.Ø. Hjortdal, Extensibility of the normo-hydrated human cornea. Acta Ophthalmol. Scand. **73**(1), 12–17 (1995)
68. C.T. McKee, J.A. Last, P. Russell, C.J. Murphy, Indentation versus tensile measurements of Young's modulus for soft biological tissues. Tissue Eng. Part B Rev. **17**(3), 155–164 (2011)
69. A.S. Kobayashi, S.L.-Y. Woo, C. Lawrence, W.A. Schlegel, Analysis of the corneo-scleral shell by the method of direct stiffness. J. Biomech. **4**(5), 323–330 (1971)
70. G.W. Nyquist, Rheology of the cornea: experimental techniques and results. Exp. Eye Res. **7** (2), 183–188 (1968)
71. H. Goldmann, Applanation tonometry, in *Glaucoma Trans Second Conf.*, ed by F.W. Newell (Josia Macy Jr Foundation, New York, 1957), pp. 167–220
72. S.-Y. Woo, A.S. Kobayashi, W.A. Schlegel, C. Lawrence, Nonlinear material properties of intact cornea and sclera. Exp. Eye Res. **14**(1), 29–39 (1972)
73. D.M. Maurice, The cornea and sclera, in *The Eye*, ed. by H. Davson (Academic Press Inc. (London) Ltd., London, 1984), p. 522
74. R.P. Vito, P.H. Carnell, Finite element based mechanical models of the cornea for pressure and indenter loading. Refract. Corneal Surg. **8**(2), 146–151 (1992)
75. M.E. Levenston, E.H. Frank, A.J. Grodzinsky, Variationally derived 3-field finite element formulations for quasistatic poroelastic analysis of hydrated biological tissues. Comput. Methods Appl. Mech. Eng. **156**(1–4), 231–246 (1998)
76. M.R. Prausnitz, J.S. Noonan, Permeability of cornea, sclera, and conjunctiva: a literature analysis for drug delivery to the eye. J. Pharm. Sci. **87**(12), 1479–1488 (1998)
77. Y. Ota, S. Mishima, D.M. Maurice, Endothelial permeability of the living cornea to fluorescein. Invest. Ophthalmol. Vis. Sci. **13**(12), 945–949 (1974)
78. L.S. Liebovitch, S. Weinbaum, A model of epithelial water transport. The corneal endothelium. Biophys. J. **35**(2), 315–338 (1981)
79. S. Hodson, C. Wigham, The permeability of rabbit and human corneal endothelium. J. Physiol. **342**(1), 409–419 (1983)
80. A. Edwards, M. Prausnitz, Predicted permeability of the cornea to topical drugs. Pharm. Res. **18**(11), 1497–1508 (2001)
81. M. Borene, V. Barocas, A. Hubel, Mechanical and cellular changes during compaction of a collagen-sponge-based corneal stromal equivalent. Ann. Biomed. Eng. **32**(2), 274–283 (2004)
82. N. Katsube, R. Wang, E. Okuma, C. Roberts, Biomechanical response of the cornea to phototherapeutic keratectomy when treated as a fluid-filled porous material. J. Refract. Surg. Thorofare NJ 1995 **18**(5), S593–S597 (2002)
83. D. Prokofiev, J. Dunec, Multiphysics model of soil phenomena near a well, in *Proc. Comsol Multiphysics User's Conf. 2005* (Boston, 2005)
84. A. Rémond, S. Naïli, T. Lemaire, Interstitial fluid flow in the osteon with spatial gradients of mechanical properties: a finite element study. Biomech. Model. Mechanobiol. **7**(6), 487–495 (2008)
85. S.D. Klyce, C.H. Dohlman, D.W. Tolpin, In vivo determination of corneal swelling pressure. Exp. Eye Res. **11**(2), 220–229 (1971)
86. B.O. Hedbys, C.H. Dohlman, A new method for the determination of the swelling pressure of the corneal stroma in vitro. Exp. Eye Res. **2**(2), 122–129 (1963)
87. S. Mishima, B.O. Hedbys, Physiology of the cornea. Int. Ophthalmol. Clin. **8**(3), 527–560 (1968)
88. T. Seiler, M. Matallana, S. Sendler, T. Bende, Does Bowman's layer determine the biomechanical properties of the cornea? Refract. Corneal Surg. **8**(2), 139–142 (1992)
89. A. Arciniegas, L.E. Amaya, Bio-structural model of the human eye. Ophthalmologica **180**(4), 207–211 (1980)
90. C.F. Burgoyne, J. Crawford Downs, A.J. Bellezza, J.-K. Francis Suh, R.T. Hart, The optic nerve head as a biomechanical structure: a new paradigm for understanding the role of IOP-

related stress and strain in the pathophysiology of glaucomatous optic nerve head damage. Prog. Retin. Eye Res. **24**(1), 39–73 (2005)

91. Y.C. Fung, *Biomechanics: Mechanical Properties of Living Tissues* (Springer, New York, 1993)

92. Y.C. Fung, S.C. Cowin, Biomechanics: mechanical properties of living tissues. J. Appl. Mech. **61**(4), 1007–1007 (1994)

93. P.B. Wilhelm, K.M. Van De Graaff, R.W. Rhees, *Schaum's Easy Outline of Human Anatomy and Physiology* (McGraw-Hill, New York, 2001)

94. J.O. Hjortdal, On the biomechanical properties of the cornea with particular reference to refractive surgery. Acta Ophthalmol. Scand. Suppl. **225**, 1–23 (1998)

95. R.F. Jones, D.M. Maurice, New methods of measuring the rate of aqueous flow in man with fluorescein. Exp. Eye Res. **5**(3), 208–220 (1966)

96. H. Wiig, Cornea fluid dynamics I: measurement of hydrostatic and colloid osmotic pressure in rabbits. Exp. Eye Res. **49**(6), 1015–1030 (1989)

97. S.D. Klyce, S.R. Russell, Numerical solution of coupled transport equations applied to corneal hydration dynamics. J. Physiol. **292**(1), 107–134 (1979)

98. S. Cronemberger, C.S. Guimarães, N. Calixto, J.M.F. Calixto, Intraocular pressure and ocular rigidity after LASIK. Arq. Bras. Oftalmol. **72**(4), 439–443 (2009)

99. W.J. Dupps Jr., M.Q. Salomão, R. Ambrósio Jr., Clinical biomechanics and the ocular response analyzer in ectatic disease, in: *Keratoconus Keratoectasia Prev. Diagn. Treat.*, ed. by M.X. Wang, T. Schroeder Swartz (SLACK Incorporated, 2010), pp. 13–28

100. I.G. Pallikaris, A.I. Dastiridou, M.K. Tsilimbaris, N.G. Karyotakis, H.S. Ginis, Ocular rigidity. Exp. Rev. Ophthalmol. **5**(3), 343–351 (2010)

101. E.T. Detorakis, I.G. Pallikaris, Ocular rigidity: biomechanical role, in vivo measurements and clinical significance. Clin. Exp. Ophthalmol. **41**(1), 73–81 (2013)

102. R. Stodtmeister, Applanation tonometry and correction according to corneal thickness. Acta Ophthalmol. Scand. **76**(3), 319–324 (1998)

103. P.J. Foster, J.-S. Wong, E. Wong, F.-G. Chen, D. Machin, P.T. Chew, Accuracy of clinical estimates of intraocular pressure in Chinese eyes. Ophthalmology **107**(10), 1816–1821 (2000)

104. M. Shimmyo, A.J. Ross, A. Moy, R. Mostafavi, Intraocular pressure, Goldmann applanation tension, corneal thickness, and corneal curvature in Caucasians, Asians, Hispanics, and African Americans. Am J. Ophthalmol. **136**(4), 603–613 (2003)

105. M. Kohlhaas, E. Spoerl, A.G. Boehm, K. Pollack, A correction formula for the real intraocular pressure after LASIK for the correction of myopic astigmatism. J. Refract. Surg. **22**(3), 263–267 (2006)

106. M.B.A. Kohlhaas, Effect of central corneal thickness, corneal curvature, and axial length on applanation tonometry. Arch. Ophthalmol. **124**(4), 471–476 (2006)

Index

A
Ablation
  deformational responses, 57
  finite element model, 58
  intrastromal ring segments, 28
  keratectasia, 58, 71
  laser, 4, 9
  scanning electron microscopy, 9, 10
  stromal bed, 57
Ablation zone, 57, 58, 70
AK. *See* Astigmatic keratotomy (AK)
ALK. *See* Automated lamellar keratoplasty
    (ALK)
Amaya, L.E., 120, 121, 129
Ametropia
  A-scan ultrasonographer, 24
  cornea, 41
  Ferrara ring, 77
  geometrical model, 41
  intrastromal ring segments, 28
  myopia, astigmatism and hypermetropia, 33
  optical correction, 91
  total refraction, 24
Anatomy
  corneal wound healing, 10
  eye globe, 127, 128
  radius of curvature and thickness, 8–9
Anisotropic model
  corneal, 3
  fibrils, 93
  isotropic hyperelastic model, 94–95
  lamella model, 94
  microstructure, 92
  mucopolysaccharides, 42, 92
  RK, 19

  stromal tissue, 59
  viscoelasticity, 18, 122
Arciniegas, A., 13, 120, 121, 129
Aristotle, 3
Astigmatic keratotomy (AK)
  ICRS, 73, 74
  incisional surgery, 1–2
  patient data, 21
Astigmatism
  corneal topography, 36
  curvature radius, 37
  heterogeneity, cornea, 96, 100–101
  intrastromal ring segments, 28, 74
  irregular, 34, 36
  Lindstrom arcuate technique, 36
  myopia, 75
  and myopia, 36
  refraction, 96
  RK, 36
  RS, 1
  segments, 96
  simulations, 96, 99, 100
Automated lamellar keratoplasty (ALK)
  computational modeling, 5
  LASIK (*see* Laser in situ keratomileusis
    (LASIK))

B
Barraquer, J., 1
Barraquer, J.I., 74
Battaglioli, J.L., 13, 118
Best-corrected visual acuity (BCVA), 77, 84
Binder, P.S., 3
Biomechanical instrumentation. *See* Tonometry